For John Johnson
Welcome to the Centre!
with best wishes.

[signature]

NY U, February 2009.

Every
Note
Counts

Every Note Counts

The Story of Nordoff-Robbins Music Therapy

Fraser Simpson

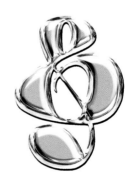

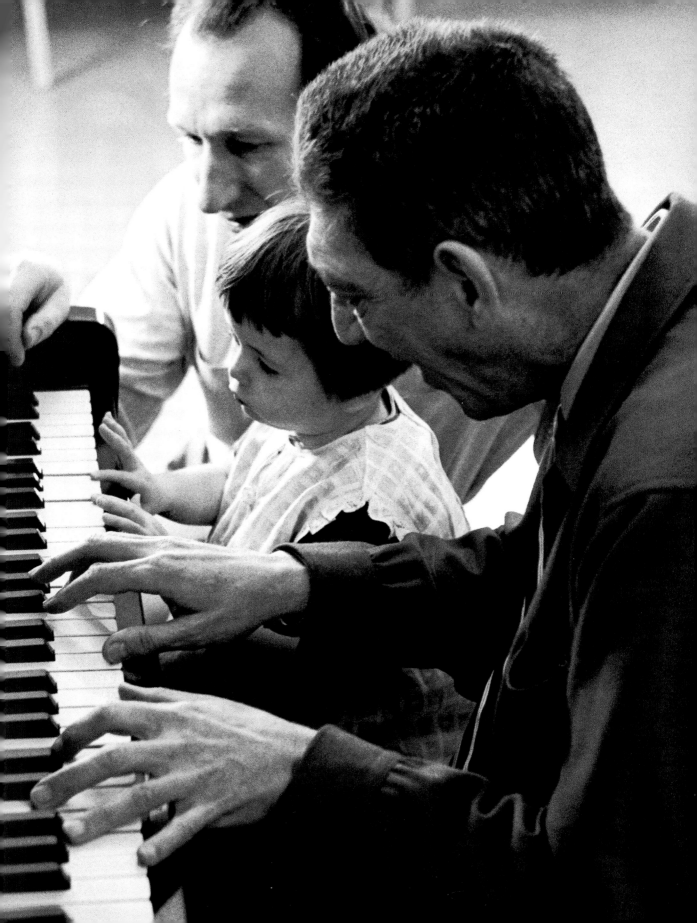

Words of Welcome

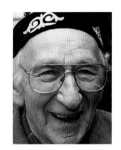

Once upon a time, there was a vision, born of a love of music and a deep concern for children with special needs, that music-making could hold as yet unknown powers as therapy for them. The vision had an inner force and direction. Creatively, carefully, in working with children, the potential that music held was explored. An effective practice of therapy matured and as it became known, dedicated individuals and professionals in the health care services took up the vision. It became a cause and gained support. With the launching of a training programme it became possible to pass on the special skills and knowledge to a new generation of therapists. More children could receive therapy. The new therapists also spread the work to address the needs of adult patients in a variety of clinics and hospitals. At this time managers and artists in the wider social world of musical enjoyment and entertainment, leading figures in the British rock music industry, became inspired by the vision of music as therapy. Their generosity, goodwill and enthusiasm abounded and through their sustained commitment the necessary financial backing was raised to build a Centre. The ever-growing success of the Centre's work led to its therapy programmes expanding widely. In three decades a musical ideal that began quietly in a children's home in the Worcestershire countryside, serving a few individuals, had expanded to become a nationwide, life-enhancing community service, serving thousands. The vision and practice also spread – as the tale will tell – to have global effect.

It is a very great honour to welcome readers to this extraordinary story. I do not need to add to the narrative for the story-telling is thoroughly researched, comprehensive and accurate, and the text vividly brought to life by well-chosen photographs that capture the past and celebrate the present.

Ultimately, this is a story of a camaraderie that embraces the immense powers of music – its powers to be a therapy that transforms lives, and its broad social powers that influence the awareness and motivation of people in the wider environment. To have personally lived the events that are recounted in these pages is an amazing reality – not only to have been involved in so many adventures of creative clinical musicianship in action with Paul Nordoff and his talented students and successors, but also to have shared the enthusiasms and experiences of countless colleagues and comrades. And to have lived to see the day when acclaimed performing musicians, household names, became public champions of music therapy has been a rare privilege indeed.

As the surviving co-founder of the approach to music therapy which is the central theme of this book I must close these words of welcome by expressing my warm appreciation to each individual whose name appears in the text for the role he or she has played, and in many instances, continues to play, in this ever unfolding story of discovery and beauty, humanity and adventure.

Clive Robbins
Founding Director
Nordoff-Robbins Center for Music Therapy, New York

Foreword

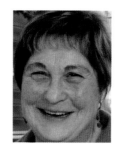

This book is dedicated to all the committed music therapists and other professionals who have contributed to the work of the Nordoff-Robbins Music Therapy charity over 32 years, and to those who have had the vision and tenacity to make this work possible through their support for the charity.

The motivation for commissioning this book followed from the death in 2002 of Sybil Beresford-Peirse, the founder and driving force of the Nordoff-Robbins Music Therapy charity in the UK. It seemed vital that the early history and development of the charity should be documented and preserved before it was lost to future generations. This book has more than fulfilled that task, and serves as an exciting record expertly woven by the author in documenting the decades of pioneering work in Nordoff-Robbins Music Therapy.

As I commend the book to you, this is also an apt opportunity for me to recognise the outstanding contribution to the charity of all the fund-raisers, and those who have voluntarily given their time and expertise so willingly to the governance of and fund-raising for the charity.

Finally, the book is a tribute to the thousands of children and adult clients and their families and carers for whom music as therapy has been a life-enhancing and healing experience.

Pauline Etkin
Managing Director
Nordoff-Robbins Music Therapy

Acknowledgements

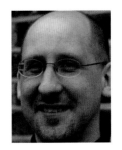

The process of writing this book has been an enormously enjoy-able one. This has been largely due to the warm co-operation of the considerable number of people whom I have consulted along the way, as well as of course the captivating interest of my subject matter. The book in essence is the biography of a uniquely inspired organisation, and in gathering and piecing together many fragments of information from different sources I have often felt as though I were completing a large jigsaw puzzle. Like any jigsaw puzzle there were times when the pieces didn't seem to quite fit together, and the process of navigating my way through conflicting accounts occasionally threatened to defeat me. The finished text represents as accurate a portrayal of events as possible within the best of my knowledge.

I am grateful first and foremost to Pauline Etkin, the Managing Director of the Nordoff-Robbins Music Therapy Charity, who conceived the idea of documenting the history of the charity, and who honoured me by inviting me to take up the task. Pauline was closely involved throughout the whole process of researching and writing, answering an endless stream of ques-tions and reading through each chapter draft as it was produced, making many useful corrections and additions.

I am also indebted to Clive Robbins, not only because the heart of the book is about his work and its legacy, but also because he gave me much support and encouragement in the task, providing me with a wealth of materials at his disposal including photographs and private correspondence

© Nordoff-Robbins Music Therapy, 2007
First published 2007
ISBN 978 1 903942 79 6

Registered in England Company No. 1514616
Registered Charity No. 280960
Nordoff-Robbins Music Therapy
2 Lissenden Gardens, London NW5 1PQ

Published by James and James (Publishers) Ltd, a member of Third Millennium Information Group
2–5 Benjamin Street, London, EC1M 5QL

JAMES
X
JAMES

Project editor: Susan Millership. Designer: Robin Farrow.
Typeset in Helvetica Neue Light Condensed 10/14.7pt
Printed and bound by Butler & Tanner, Frome, Somerset.

with Sybil Beresford-Peirse, answering my many enquiries always promptly, and reading through various drafts and revisions of the text.

Thirdly, my thanks are due to Sam Alder, who retires this year after ten years as Chairman of Nordoff-Robbins' Board of Governors and 32 years of service for the charity as a founding member of the fund-raising committee. He warmly supported the project from the outset, advised on many aspects of the work and was closely involved in bringing it to publication.

James & James Publishers offered very favourable terms for publishing this book and it has been a great pleasure to work with its Managing Director, Hamish MacGibbon, Project Editor, Susan Millership, and Designer, Robin Farrow. I would like to thank them for the superb quality of all aspects of their work, and for their patient tolerance of delays in assembling drafts of the text and photographic materials.

I would also like to thank the many people with whom I conducted tape-recorded interviews for this project between 2002 and 2004, and who generously and enthusiastically shared their time and knowledge with me. Many of them also later scoured the text for accuracy, in portion or full, and added further insight. Occasional unsourced quotations in the text are drawn from these interviews. The people I interviewed were:

Sam Alder, Gary Ansdell, Merete Birkebæk, Alyson Carter, Jack Dobbs, Jean Eisler, Pauline Etkin, Rosemary Evans, Jane Gibson, Nick Hampton, Robin Howat, Althea Mapplebeck, Selina Mapplebeck, Andrew Miller, Mercédès Pavlicevic, Jacqueline Robarts, Willie Robertson, Clive Robbins, Steve Stanton, Malcolm Troup, Rachel Verney and Sarah Verney Caird.

A number of other people also kindly assisted me, sometimes investing a considerable amount of time, often putting useful literature or photographs at my disposal, and checking portions of the text. They are: Mary Abbotson, Ken Aigen, Julie Allis, Sandra Brown, The Earl of Bradford, Matthew Dixon, Gemma Fleet, Yid-Ee Goh, Claire Hay, Audrey Hoare, Nancy Jarratt, John Marshall and his team at JM International, Anthony Mapplebeck, Ivy McGeorge, Joe Meaney, Margaret Midson, Julian Morgenstern, Nicky O'Neill, Lutz Neugebauer, Helen Patey, James Robertson, Enid Rowe, Julie Sutton, Alan Turry, Sheila Tyler (sadly deceased) and Oksana Zharinova-Sanderson.

Finally, I owe thanks to my other friends and colleagues within the Nordoff-Robbins Charity, as well as Nordoff-Robbins colleagues abroad, too many to name individually, for their warm support, interest, encouragement, assistance and innumerable helpful ideas while this project has been underway.

Fraser Simpson, May 2007

Picture Credits

Every effort has been made to trace the source of photo-graphic material used in this book and to seek the necessary permission to reproduce it. Any omission of acknowledge-ment is inadvertent and will be corrected, where attention is drawn, in any future publications. Thanks are due to clients and their families for permission to print pictures. Photographs are credited to the following persons and organ-isations: Sandra Brown *70 (bottom left), 88 (Julie Sutton, Gary Ansdell, Rachel Verney, Donald Wetherick)*; Matthew Dixon *88 (Nicky O'Neill, Simon Procter)*; Robin Farrow *4, 76 (bottom), 88 (Mercédès Pavlicevic, Jacqueline Robarts), 94-95*; Peter Higginbotham *43*; Arnold Johnson *88 (Judith Nockolds)*; John Marshall *6, 9, 12, 15, 17, 19, 20-21, 22-23, 24-25, 32, 44, 53 (right), 56, 68-69, 80 (inset), 88 (Helen Patey, Sandra Brown), 91 (lower three), 92-93, 108, 110-111, 112 (bottom), 113 (top)*; Martikainen, Majalampi, Suomi-Finland *2-3, 34 (top), 35 (top)*; Chris Nichols *102*; Ulf Nilson, Berlingske Tidende *37 (top)*; Barry Plummer front cover, *10-11, 16, 38, 47, 48, 49, 50-51, 52-53, 60-61, 64-65, 66, 67 (left), 72-73, 79, 80-81 (large), 84, 87, 98, 113 (bottom)*; Clive Robbins *27, 28, 34-35 (bottom), 37 (bottom), 101*; Leo Sorel *33, 100*; The Medical Illustration Department, Merton & Sutton NHS Trust *65 (right)*.

All photographs in this book are protected by copyright and may not be reproduced without permission from copyright holders. The copyright holder for all photographs is Nordoff-Robbins Music Therapy (UK) except for the following: The International Trust for Nordoff-Robbins Music Therapy *2-3, 27, 28, 29, 31, 32, 33, 34-35, 37, 100, 101, 107*; Nordoff-Robbins Music Therapy Australia *104, 105*; Nordoff-Robbins Music Therapy in Scotland *96 (all)*; Mary Abbotson *78*; City University, London *71*; Herdecke Hospital, Germany *103*; Peter Higginbotham/ www.workhouses.org.uk *43*; New York University *102*; unknown *50 (left), 67 (right)*.

Contents

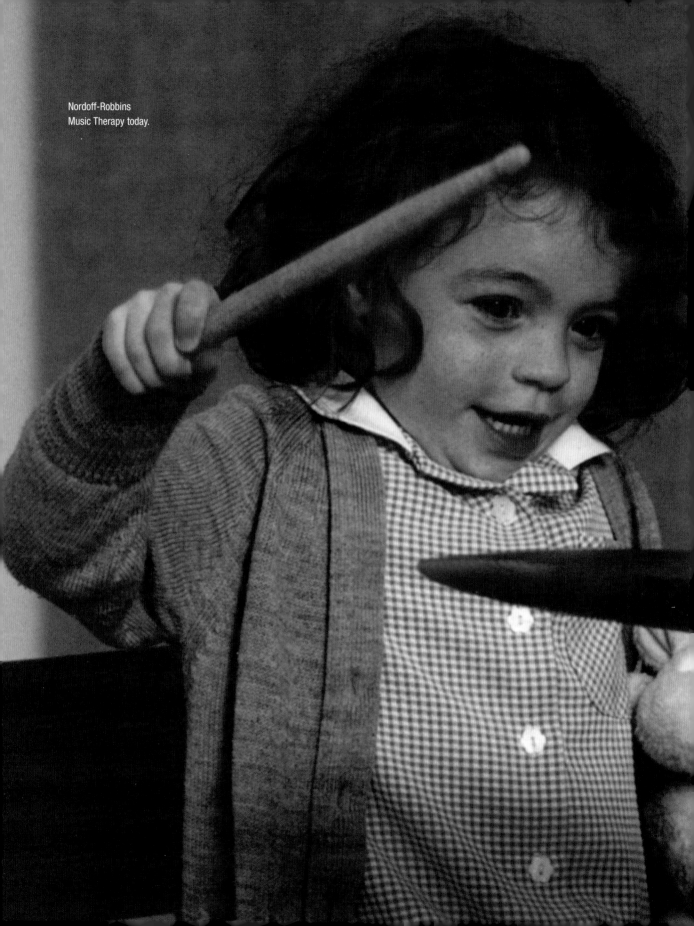

Nordoff-Robbins
Music Therapy today.

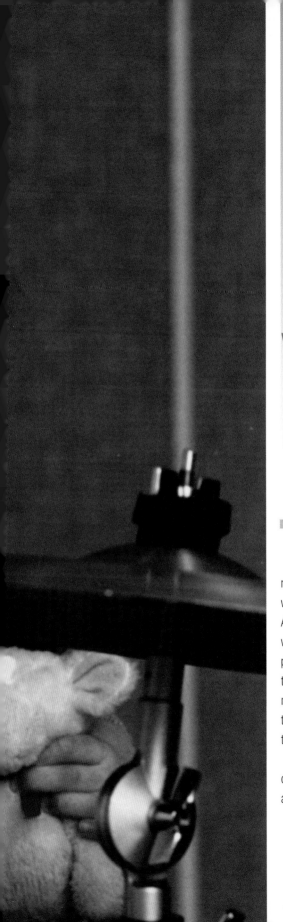

Welcome to Nordoff-Robbins

The name of Nordoff-Robbins is known today to countless people in association with the art of healing through music. A national charity established in 1976, Nordoff-Robbins Music Therapy has earned the respect and support of professional musicians from the popular and classical worlds, eminent physicians, psychologists, educationalists and many others. At an embryonic stage of its development, Nordoff-Robbins Music Therapy was fortunate to win the support of the rock music industry, and this patronage has made a fundamental contribution to the continued growth of the charity; today Nordoff-Robbins is lucky enough to remain as one of the main charities supported by the music industry. This support remains essential for the charity to continue to operate, and provide over 30,000 music therapy sessions at over 50 locations nationwide each year.

What is music therapy? Who goes to see a music therapist? What happens during a music therapy session? These are just some of the questions that are asked frequently of those who undertake or support the work of Nordoff-

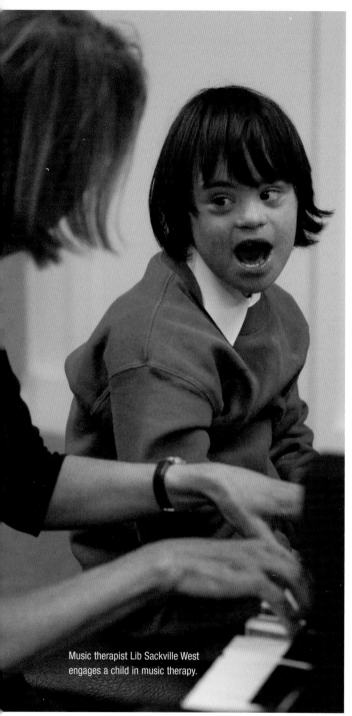

Music therapist Lib Sackville West engages a child in music therapy.

Robbins Music Therapy. Instinctively, no one doubts the therapeutic properties of music, but how does music therapy differ from music itself? Although music therapy is based on the power of music, it has an agenda: it is music-making with

> The overall aim of Music Therapy is to actively engage individuals in their own growth . . . bringing them from isolation into active participation in the world.

goals that reach *beyond* music. In the words of Clive Robbins, one of the original founders of Nordoff-Robbins Music Therapy: 'The overall aim of Music Therapy is to actively engage individuals in their own growth, development and behavioural change and for them to transfer musical and non-musical skills to other aspects of their life, bringing them from isolation into active participation in the world.'

Music has an effect that words cannot achieve, as every music lover knows. Just as a textual analysis of a Beethoven symphony is no substitute for the symphony itself, so a book about music therapy cannot satisfactorily communicate the power of music therapy. This book aims only to whet the appetite of those who would explore further, and to inform of the remarkable history of this inspirational music therapy charity.

Music therapy is conducted by registered health professionals trained to degree level who, first and foremost, are highly skilled musicians. These people have learned how to use musical improvisation to draw others into shared music-making; the creative processes which result from this interaction have been observed to have a dramatic effect on a person's ability to function in his or her world. Many individuals who come to music therapy have an identifiable disability, illness or trauma which limits their range of experience or capabilities. A toddler displaying autistic symptoms, a young woman with Down's syndrome, a middle-aged man with

The basic elements of music are manifested physiologically in our bodies . . . This is why music therapy has the potential to help almost anyone.

chronic mental health problems, a motorcyclist brain-damaged in an accident, a frail, elderly woman with advanced dementia – these and many others are referred to music therapy. Sometimes people decide to visit a music therapist, simply intrigued by the idea that making music with another human being might yield them insights into their inner being. The common thread that connects these individuals is that peculiar, universal responsiveness to music that is the privilege of humanity. For the basic elements of music – tempo, rhythm, melody – are manifested physiologically in our bodies: when we organise them, as we do in music, we are pleased, excited, calmed, enlivened. Music calls to us, orders us, and literally brings us together. This is why music therapy has the potential to help almost anyone.

The work of Nordoff-Robbins today: therapy, training and research

Nordoff-Robbins Music Therapy is a UK-based charity offering services throughout the country. It has a tripartite directive: to provide therapy, training and research. This work is conducted at the charity's National Headquarters in Kentish Town, north

Kalvin

Kalvin was an animated nine-year-old, with severe learning disabilities and autism, but the main reason that his school referred him for music therapy was his challenging behaviour. Kalvin's music therapists were subjected to many of his habitual misdemeanours as he spat (on the instruments as well as directly at the therapists), stripped off his clothes and leapt about the room, yelling. He avoided engaging in any music-making and evaded eye contact.

Kalvin attended weekly individual sessions for three years. The first significant development came when Kalvin began to lie on the floor quietly for extended periods, his attention caught by the music played in response to his movements and sounds. This led to some sustained eye contact and intermittent exploration of small instruments offered to him. When these minimal musical sounds were reflected back to him, Kalvin showed amusement and sometimes delight. He began to produce sustained and tuneful notes with his voice, and approached the side drum and cymbal boldly.

Progress was patchy because moments of significant development were often followed by a withdrawal into previous behaviours. It seemed that Kalvin found it threatening to experience direct interaction with the therapists. But little by little he responded increasingly to the musical 'demands' made of him, giving rise to extended imitative work and playful turn-taking with the therapists. His behaviour improved, and in the final sessions Kalvin reached a level of expressive communication that would have been unimaginable at the beginning.

In music therapy Kalvin was accepted for who he was. His latent abilities and capacity to relate were drawn out of him through his responsiveness to music. At the end his appreciative school reported a marked improvement in Kalvin's ability to engage positively in the classroom, with adults and with other children.

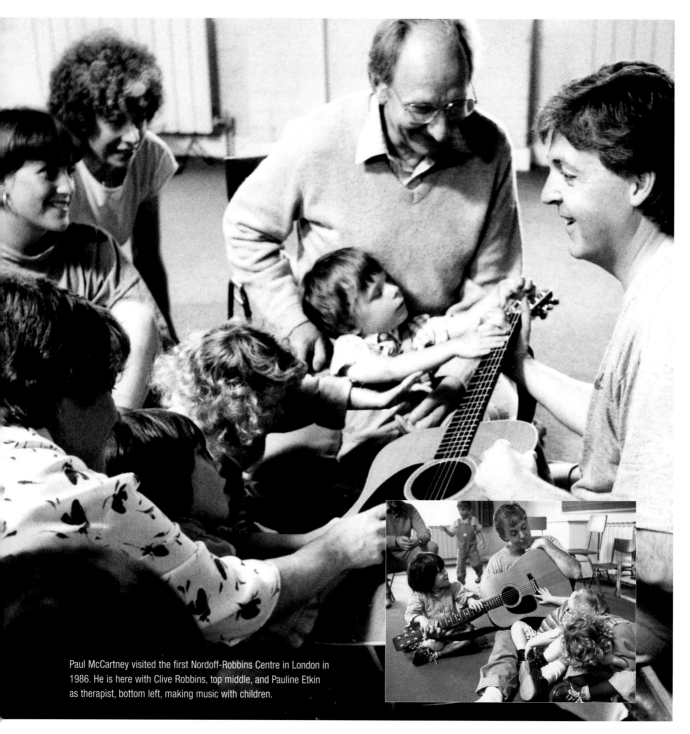

Paul McCartney visited the first Nordoff-Robbins Centre in London in
1986. He is here with Clive Robbins, top middle, and Pauline Etkin
as therapist, bottom left, making music with children.

London, which houses the largest music therapy centre in the world, as well as in various regional Units and workplaces around the UK.

The therapy work itself is the central object of the charity's existence, and this work is made possible by the rigorous two-year training for musicians to become qualified music therapists. As a young profession in a demanding public service economy, music therapy needs continually to make its effectiveness explicit and demonstrable; the Nordoff-Robbins charity takes this obligation seriously and funds a research department based at the National Headquarters. All this is facilitated through fund-raising activities and the generous support of the music industry.

At the Nordoff-Robbins Music Therapy National Centre up to 200 children, adolescents and adults receive music therapy every week, referred by local schools, parents, GPs, psychologists and other professionals (or by self-referral). The Centre is equipped with facilities for three sessions to take place simultaneously in separate, soundproofed rooms. Three therapy rooms are equipped with an observation booth and one-way mirror, which allows music therapy trainees to observe sessions – a vital element of their training. Further rooms enable therapists and students to review their sessions recorded on video or audio. The Centre has a spacious conference hall seating 150 (which can also be used as a further therapy room) – a wonderful resource which is frequently used by the music therapy profession* making the Centre a focal point for professional activity and development. There are also specialist library resources, teaching space for the training programme and student facilities.

There are two Nordoff-Robbins Music Therapy Master's degree training programmes in the UK: one based at the National Centre and validated by City University, and the other at Queen Margaret University in Edinburgh. A third training programme in Community Music Therapy is scheduled to begin in Manchester in 2008. Each year an average of 16

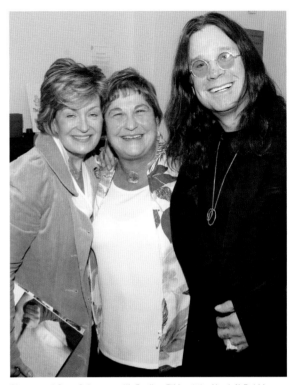

Sharon and Ozzy Osbourne with Pauline Etkin at the Nordoff-Robbins National Centre in London, 2006.

proficient musicians (six in London and ten in Edinburgh) begin an intensive two-year programme that teaches them to meet, through musical improvisation, the many pathologies and conditions which music therapists encounter in clinical practice on a daily basis. Students receive individualised tuition in improvisation techniques and keyboard skills, observe sessions and begin closely supervised clinical work. They receive their own confidential personal therapy and attend background lectures in psychiatry, disability, child development and other specialist areas. They learn skills of assessment and documentation, casework presentation, multidisciplinary teamwork and research methods. The training in London was the first permanent Nordoff-Robbins training programme to be established in the world. It has

* Music therapy became a registered UK profession in June 1999, and is registered with the Health Professions Council; this was the culmination of a process that took many years, and in which Pauline Etkin, Managing Director of Nordoff-Robbins, was closely involved from an early stage.

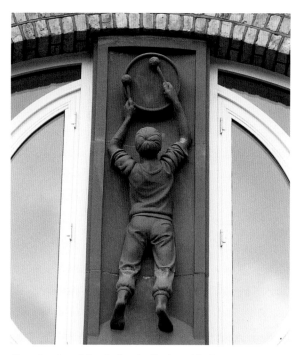

Above, facade sculpture by Douglas Binnie, architect.
Facing page, Beresford-Peirse House, Lissenden Gardens – the Nordoff-Robbins Music Therapy National Centre in Kentish Town, north London.

Meeting the child where he is

The art of music can be consciously directed towards the non-communicating or severely physically handicapped child, to penetrate the barriers set up by his illness and to motivate him to take part in inter-responsive activity. The very form and structure inherent in music can bring a meaningful sense of order and security to the mentally or emotionally disabled. When working with an individual child the therapist uses a creative dynamic approach, improvising at the piano and vocally, seeking to meet the child where he is, in his frustration, rage, anxiety, apathy or sadness, and to give him the experience of his mood being met and understood in the music. Improvised music can respond immediately to any change in the mood of the child, can pick up the slightest clue at the moment it occurs, engage and develop it, so leading the child into a working situation.

Sybil Beresford-Peirse,
Director and Founder of Nordoff-Robbins
Music Therapy, London, 1974–1991

been validated since 1983 by City University, and many students have come from abroad to train. Since the programme's inception in 1974, there have been 210 successful graduates to date.

The Charity's research department makes a major contribution to the profile of music therapy research in the UK. It ensures that students on the Master's programme enter the profession not only as practitioners, but as researchers, equipped to undertake research in their chosen field of work, as employers increasingly require. A number of research projects have been completed in recent years, or are under way in the department, with accompanying publications: an 80-page guide, *Presenting the Evidence: A Guide for Music Therapists Responding to the Demands of Clinical Effectiveness and Evidence-Based Practice* (2004), was

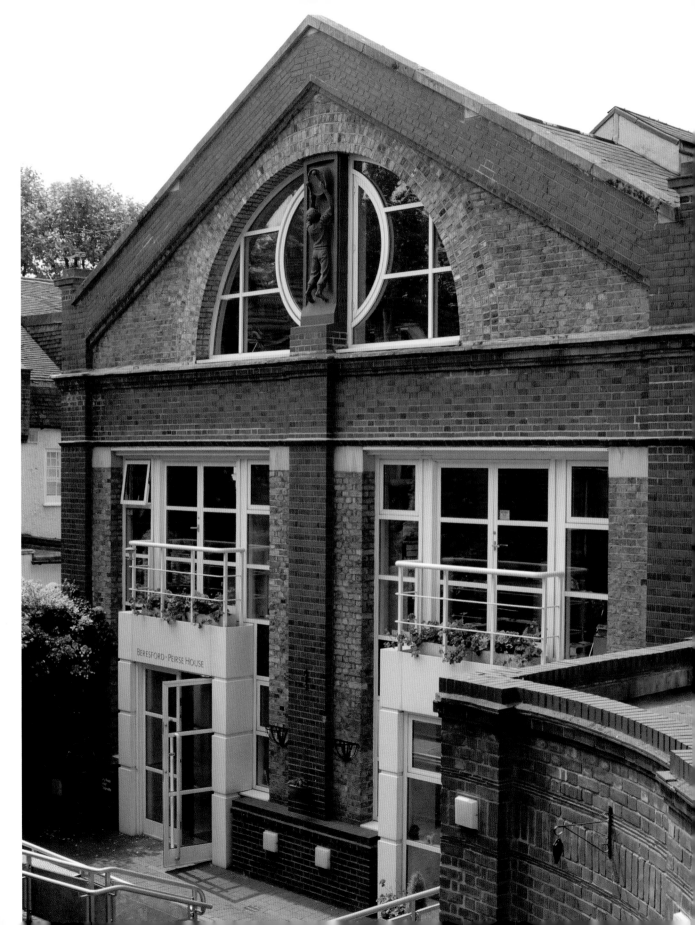

Rebecca

Tiny and frail, Rebecca, aged 33, had lived in institutional care from the age of six. Her multiple disabilities from birth included cerebral palsy and severe visual impairment, which left her with very restricted movement and apparently oblivious to her environment. She developed no speech or noticeable understanding of language. Rebecca regularly cried for no clear reason and was often moved into a separate room to avoid disturbing other residents.

With such extensive disability, Rebecca could participate in very little, but when visited by the music therapist, she revealed a surprising sensitivity to music in the first session: Rebecca's habitual wailing tuned to the key of the soft piano chords played by the therapist, and when the therapist sang back similar sounds a kind of musical conversation developed. By the end of that session Rebecca's voice quality had changed, and her wailing had turned to singing.

Rebecca was seen regularly in music therapy for the next two years. After only five sessions her ward manager observed that Rebecca cried much less and was able to spend more time with the other residents. Rebecca's music therapist found that her vocal sounds initially became stronger as she realised the expressive possibilities of the therapy and was able to give voice to her anger. The therapist accompanied this with harsh music that matched Rebecca's tone quality. Over a period of months this new expressive ability increased and she was able to express a whole variety of moods, from sadness and despair to contentment and humour.

After nearly two years the ward manager reported that Rebecca now used her voice more flexibly and communicatively outside the sessions; she showed greater response when greeted or touched and was beginning to use different sounds to indicate different needs.

The sessions by now had developed a peaceful quality that had not been present at the beginning, and the music was often light and gentle in mood, with playful laughter from Rebecca.

published in response to requests from therapists in Nordoff-Robbins outreach venues. A major international four-year research collaboration between the Nordoff-Robbins Music Therapy Centre, Sogn og Fjordane University College, Sandane (Norway) and the University of Pretoria (South Africa) also commenced in 2004. One of the most exciting recent developments has been the inauguration of an MPhil/PhD research degree programme, validated by City University, and launched in January 2006. In conjunction with this the Nordoff-Robbins Research Ethics Committee has been established to review any research associated with the organisation and to ensure that appropriate ethical standards are upheld. The new PhD programme is undoubtedly set to develop the international profile of the Charity, which can justifiably be regarded as a global beacon for music therapy activity in the 21st century.

The therapy work at the Centre is reflected and extended throughout the UK via a network of regional Nordoff-Robbins units and projects, where hundreds of people receive music therapy each week.

At no time has the income ever been guaranteed: each year it is raised from scratch.

Funding

Nordoff-Robbins Music Therapy is a registered charity (No. 280960), that needs to raise almost £3 million a year to continue to operate and grow. Although the scope of its services is enhanced by the financial contribution of those service users who are able to pay for their therapy, the enduring support and dedication of the Nordoff-Robbins fund-raisers,

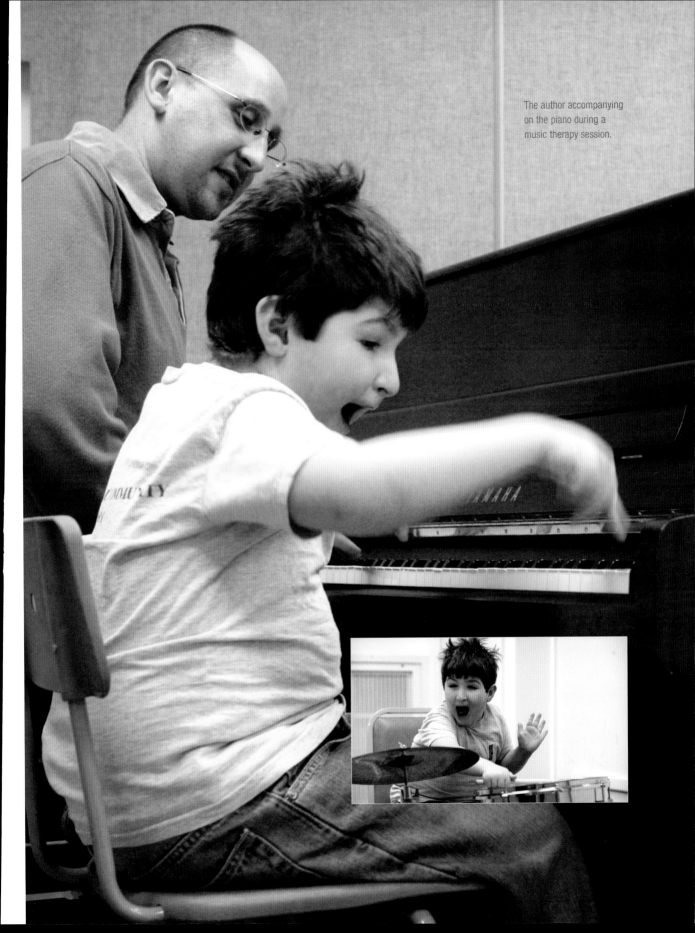

The author accompanying on the piano during a music therapy session.

The O₂ Silver Clef Lunch

The 30th Silver Clef Lunch sponsored by O₂ was a particularly sensational event, with 830 people gathering at the Inter-Continental Hotel on the edge of Hyde Park. The colourful mix of celebrity faces, music business luminaries and representatives of dozens of corporate sponsors, each paid several hundred pounds to attend. Hosted by Chris Evans, it began with a gourmet lunch, after which the mother of a young boy currently receiving music therapy at the Centre gave a moving account of how music therapy had helped her son, illustrated with short video extracts. This opportunity to hear about the work from parents is an important feature of fund-raising events.

Then it was time for the auction. Seventeen donated prizes fetched some astounding prices: a custom-built Fender Guitar, signed by artists at the 1990 Knebworth concert, sold for £52,000. A sculpture of U2 made by Laura Lian, and signed by all four band members, went for £20,000. Funk musician Jay Kay of Jamiroquai auctioned off Raymond Weil watches (including his own custom-designed one), fetching a total of £44,000. Guests bid for some great trips – to fly business class to Las Vegas and see Elton John on his Red Piano Tour, meeting Sir Elton afterwards; to take 20 friends for dinner in the historic cellars of Berry Brothers & Rudd, hosted by TV presenter Michael Parkinson.

An award ceremony followed, with prizes for rock legends The Who and U2, as well as for newer acts Lemar, McFly, Razorlight, Natasha Bedingfield and Katherine Jenkins. The awards were sponsored by corporate supporters of Nordoff-Robbins, and received in person by the stars. Finally, there was a raffle, with great prizes, including £500 vouchers for Waterstone's and HMV, and a spa holiday in Dubai. This fantastic afternoon raised a record-breaking £700,000 for Nordoff-Robbins Music Therapy.

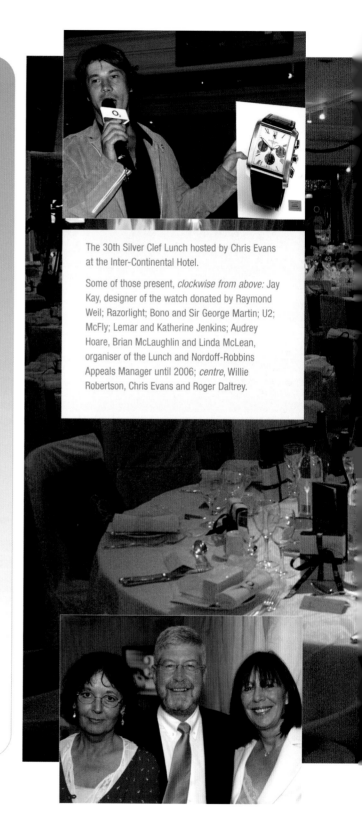

The 30th Silver Clef Lunch hosted by Chris Evans at the Inter-Continental Hotel.

Some of those present, *clockwise from above:* Jay Kay, designer of the watch donated by Raymond Weil; Razorlight; Bono and Sir George Martin; U2; McFly; Lemar and Katherine Jenkins; Audrey Hoare, Brian McLaughlin and Linda McLean, organiser of the Lunch and Nordoff-Robbins Appeals Manager until 2006; *centre,* Willie Robertson, Chris Evans and Roger Daltrey.

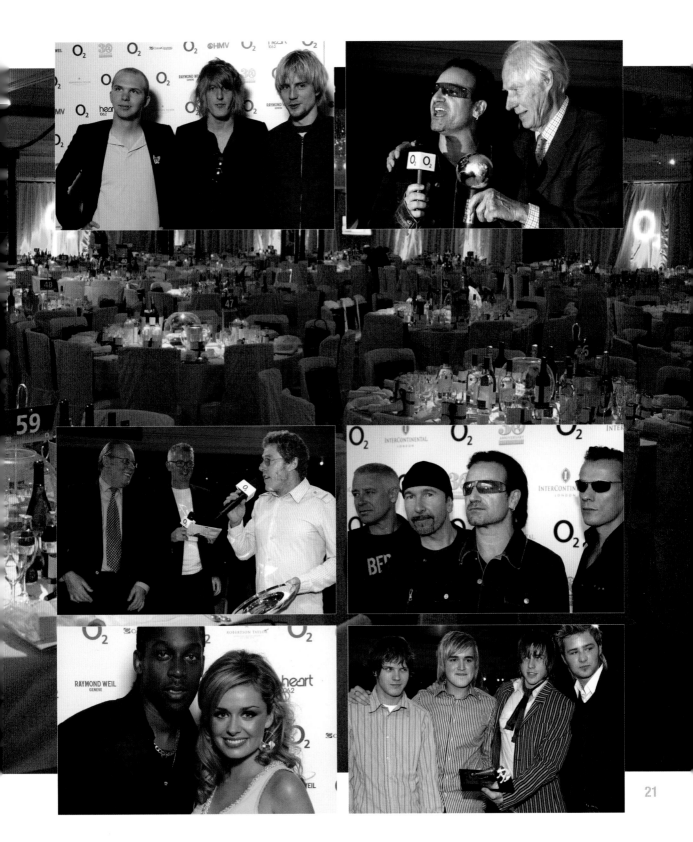

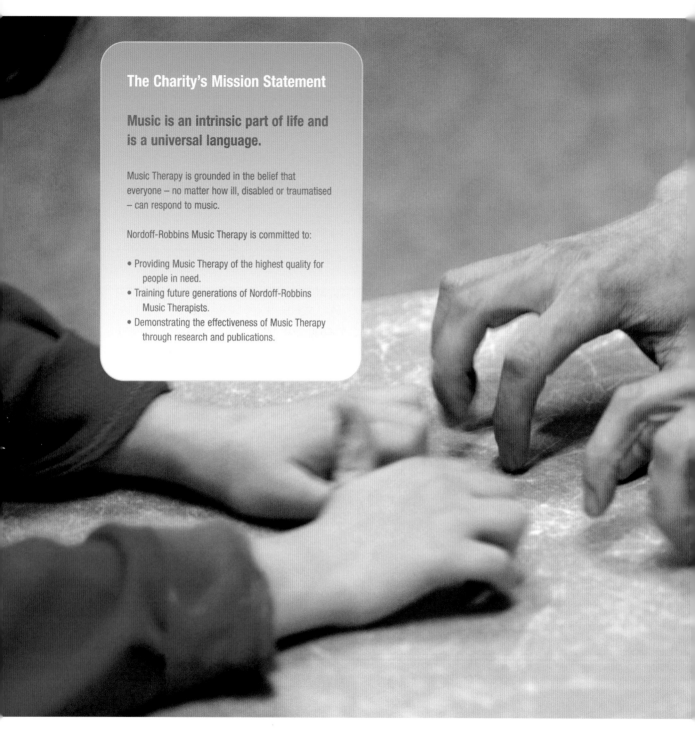

The Charity's Mission Statement

Music is an intrinsic part of life and is a universal language.

Music Therapy is grounded in the belief that everyone – no matter how ill, disabled or traumatised – can respond to music.

Nordoff-Robbins Music Therapy is committed to:

- Providing Music Therapy of the highest quality for people in need.
- Training future generations of Nordoff-Robbins Music Therapists.
- Demonstrating the effectiveness of Music Therapy through research and publications.

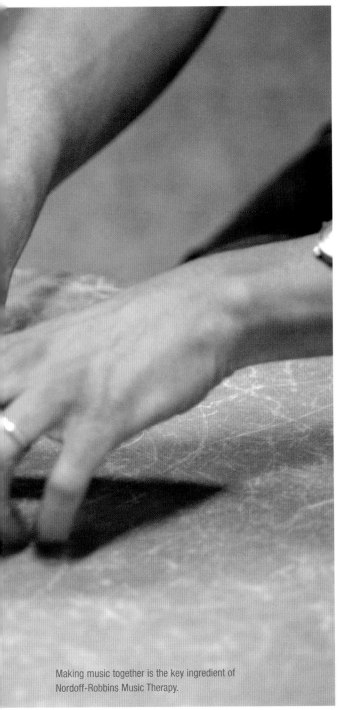

Making music together is the key ingredient of
Nordoff-Robbins Music Therapy.

donors and volunteers are critical for the continued development of Nordoff-Robbins. The charity has always ensured
that the highest possible percentage of funds raised reach
children and adults in need. The achievement is all the more
remarkable because at no time has the income ever been
guaranteed: each year it is raised from scratch.

The sums raised each year highlight the way in which the
work of Nordoff-Robbins reaches into people's hearts, particularly those with a love of music and a concern for people in
need. As the vision has grown, so the funds have risen to
meet it. The Silver Clef Lunch is an annual event honouring
musicians with all proceeds going to Nordoff-Robbins Music
Therapy. The first Lunch in 1976 raised £12,000, and by the
end of 1978 the net profit of all fund-raising activities had
topped £100,000. The Lunch went on to raise £65,345 in
1984, £200,000 in 1988, £400,000 in 2002, and an
amazing £700,000 in 2005 (the 30th anniversary of the
Lunch). The support of the rock music industry has been
constant throughout, and without this the charity would not
be where it is today. The Silver Clef Awards have become
prestigious honours bestowed only on musicians who have
reached the pinnacle of their profession.

The Silver Clef Lunch has been a phenomenal success story
for several reasons. First, of course, it is driven by the music
therapy work itself, the potency of which captures the heart
and the imagination. Secondly, it was fortuitous for Nordoff-
Robbins that in the mid-1970s there was no other major
charity being supported by the rock industry. The timing was
brilliant; and its ideal of transforming people's lives through
music was one to which musicians could relate easily.

The Silver Clef Lunches are extremely enjoyable, due not
least to the celebrities who attend (the golden rule being that
winners must receive their awards in person). They are events
where contacts are made and maintained, both business and
social, and people feel glad to be part of the music industry's
social calendar. Finally, the event's enduring success can also

be attributed to the fact that the Fund-Raising Committee is managed by highly skilled, dedicated individuals who are experts in their field.

The generous support of corporate sponsors has also given rise to other events in the Nordoff-Robbins fund-raising calendar. The HMV Football Extravaganza at the Grosvenor House Hotel began in 1996, using the same recipe of high-profile awards and an auction; it now rivals the Silver Clef Lunch and raised £608,000 in 2006. Other events include the Sandown Park Race Day, the Six Nations Rugby Championship Dinner, the Women of the Year Awards, the Christmas Carol Service and the Music Industry Trusts Dinner. There have been stunning one-off events, the biggest of which was the amazing televised Knebworth concert in June 1990, which raised the millions needed to build the National Centre at Kentish Town. Nordoff-Robbins Music Therapy strikes a chord with music fans everywhere; its appeal is universal, and therein lies its remarkable strength.

Next we turn back the clock nearly 50 years and enter an unassuming school in the Worcestershire countryside, where Nordoff-Robbins Music Therapy had its beginnings.

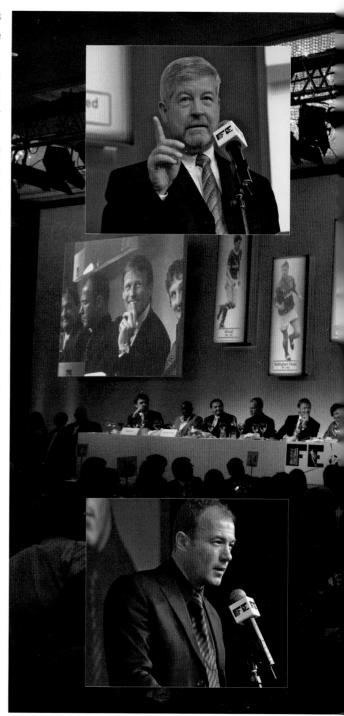

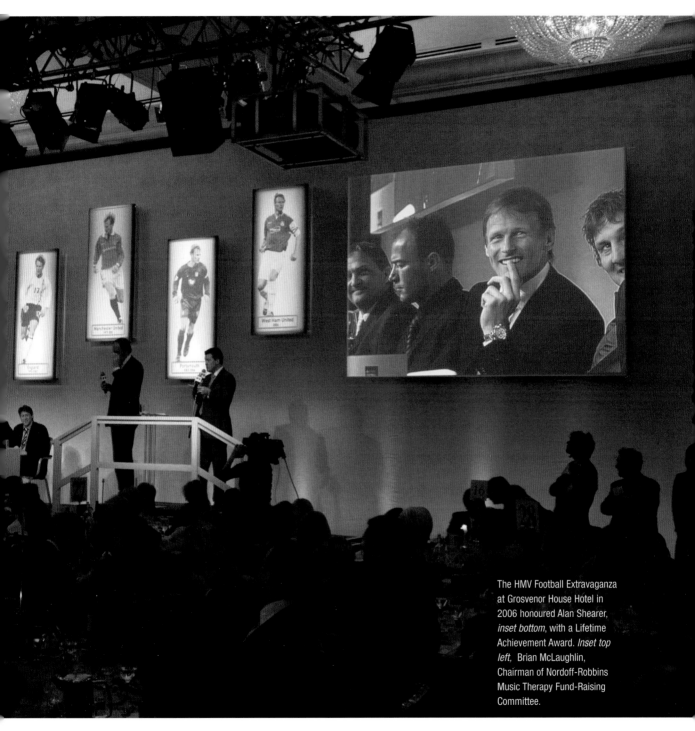

The HMV Football Extravaganza at Grosvenor House Hotel in 2006 honoured Alan Shearer, *inset bottom*, with a Lifetime Achievement Award. *Inset top left,* Brian McLaughlin, Chairman of Nordoff-Robbins Music Therapy Fund-Raising Committee.

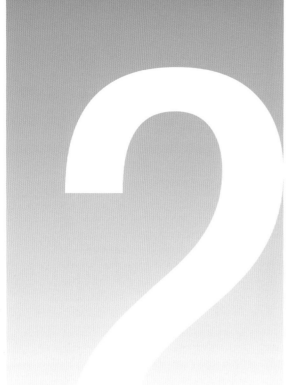

Here I am in Europe with a trunk full of music trying to get a symphony performed and here is a musician using music to bring a child into speech. There is no doubt in my mind which is the more important.

Paul Nordoff

Origin of the Work

Paul Nordoff in Europe: 1958

When American musician Paul Nordoff took a sabbatical in 1958, to visit Europe and bring his music to a wider audience, it proved to be an unexpected, life-changing experience. Professionally, the trip was not a success: despite his distinguished credentials, he encountered indifference and even some hostility from the European musical establishment. But in London he was fascinated by a lecture at Rudolf Steiner House, given by the eminent Austrian anthroposophist, Dr Karl Koenig (1902–66), who described a programme of treatment for children with cerebral palsy, combining light, colour and movement, accompanied by specially composed music. Shortly afterwards, while visiting an anthroposophical home in Germany, he observed a musician, Dr Julius Knierim, working with children, using a lyre. One girl was encouraged to pluck the strings and simultaneously formulate words, and by this method she could put together an entire sentence. Paul later recalled his reaction: 'Here I am in Europe with a trunk full of music trying to get a symphony performed and here is a musician using music to bring a child into speech. There is no doubt in my mind which is the more important.'

Sunfield Children's Homes

Paul Nordoff also visited Sunfield Children's Home in Worcestershire, having met the Director, Michael Wilson, in the USA the previous year. Sunfield, in the small village of Clent, was an anthroposophical foundation, established in the 1930s, which became one of the leading 'Curative Educational Communities' in the UK. It provided for about 75 developmentally delayed and multiply-disabled children, aged 4–17. Michael Wilson was an accomplished violinist and music played an important part at Sunfield.

Four years earlier, in 1954, Clive Robbins and his wife had joined the community at Sunfield, drawn by the atmosphere of gentle care, sincerity and good humour, the beautiful natural surroundings, the creativity and the essence of the community-based existence. Clive had never heard of anthroposophy before, but as an apprentice teacher he studied the tradition in depth. Living in this community, where spiritual beliefs were lived out as values, gave him the first profoundly fulfilling experience of his life.

However, as time went on Clive grew disheartened about some of the most disabled children, who bore tragic lives of distress and self-injury, and appeared unreachable. Clive became uneasy and wondered if the thinking and practice of the community required modernising. His wish was answered partially in 1957, when Dr Herbert Geuter (the son of one of the co-founders of Sunfield) joined the staff as Director of

Anthroposophy

Anthroposophy, an influential European movement of social, cultural and spiritual renewal, was founded around the turn of the 20th century by the Austrian philosopher and teacher, Rudolf Steiner (1861–1925). Literally the 'wisdom of man' (Greek: *anthropos* = man; *sophia* = wisdom), anthroposophy emerged as a contemporary spiritual path, based on the scientific study of the spiritual nature of humanity and the cosmos. Arousing wide and often controversial interest, Steiner's voluminous writings, lectures and practical initiatives have had a profound influence worldwide, in many diverse spheres of activity, including education, special education, medicine and health care, agriculture, architecture, the arts, industry and ethical investment. Anthroposophical work has flourished consistently, and its noble intentions for humanity – creativity, healing, freedom and responsibility – have been powerful shaping forces in the development of much contemporary thought and activity.

Dr Herbert Geuter, Clive and Paul's mentor.

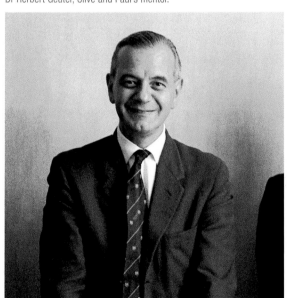

Research and became a very influential figure for Clive, both personally and professionally, bringing to Sunfield a clearer and more authentic interpretation of Steiner's work (see box).

Paul Nordoff's visit the following year was a further revelation for Clive. Paul gave an evening concert in the beautiful, wood-panelled hall at Sunfield, and Clive listened spellbound from the balcony above as Paul sat at the grand piano, singing some of his settings of poetry by E. E. Cummings, Edna St Vincent Millay and Conrad Aiken. Paul's presence was riveting and Clive later remembered the impact of the concert as 'the most living and marvellous musical experience of my life'. He remembered thinking: 'This is a sun among men. This is a man who radiates warmth and a certain strong regard for human life.'

Paul, for his part, was deeply impressed with Sunfield. He returned to America enthused, and the following year (1959)

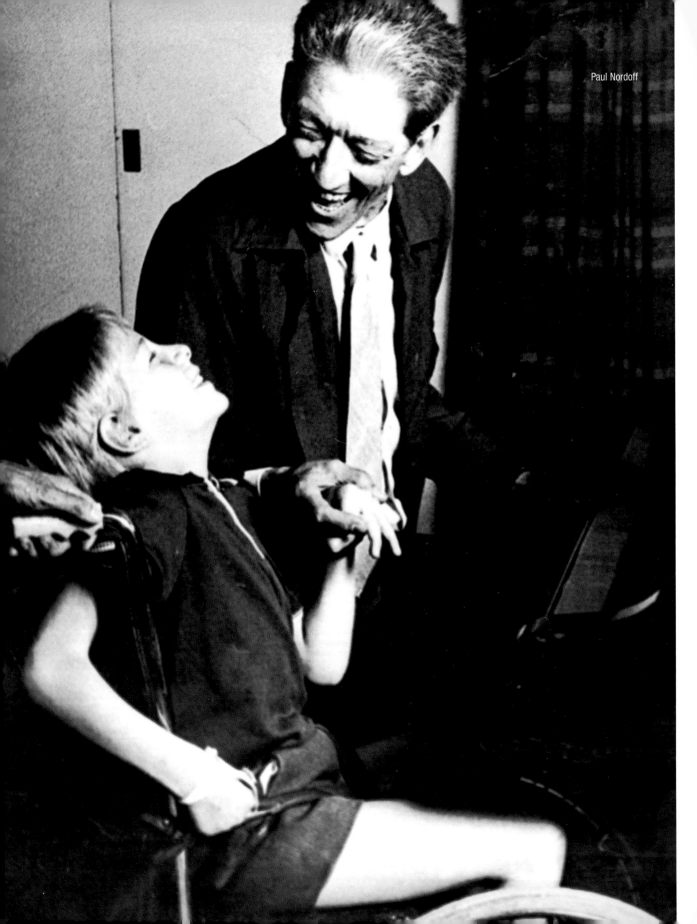

Paul Nordoff

Paul Nordoff, 1909–77

Paul Nordoff was a renowned and distinguished musician in the USA. Born in Philadelphia on 4 June 1909, he studied at the Philadelphia Conservatory of Music and the Juilliard School, winning prizes and fellowships in both performance and composition, before being appointed Head of Composition at the Philadelphia Conservatory in 1938. He was Assistant Professor of Composition at Michigan State University from 1945 and Assistant Professor of Music at Bard College, New York, from 1949 and Professor at Bard College from 1953 to 1959. In addition to his educational responsibilities, he was active as a pianist and composer, writing symphonies, concertos, chamber, vocal and stage works. Paul was awarded an honorary doctorate from Combs College of Music, Philadelphia, in 1958.

Unlike the mainstream American avant-garde of his generation, Paul's compositional style was tonal and lyrical, often written within traditional structures. He loved the Broadway musical tradition and his own compositions show the deep influence of this style. He believed that contemporary classical music should not become the preserve of an intellectual elite, divorced from the tastes and loves of the populace, but should aspire to answer the musical needs of society at large. Such views were to play an important role in his vision of how music might be used as a therapeutic medium.

In the 1940s, alongside his work as a professional musician, Paul developed a deep interest in anthroposophy, leading him, in 1946, to join Threefold Farm, an anthroposophical community in Spring Valley, New York. He lived there with his wife Sabina, a Broadway dancer and teacher of eurhythmy (an art of movement developed in anthroposophy), together with their three children, Anthony, Sylvia and Guy.

Paul Nordoff first encountered the use of music as therapy during his European tour in 1958. Fascinated by the possibilities he glimpsed in this work, he resigned his academic position and dedicated the rest of his life to the development and establishment of music therapy.

he boldly resigned his professorship in order to spend a year at Sunfield, exploring the therapeutic potential of music. Herbert ('Hep') Geuter was delighted to have him, as he was also beginning to look at the application of the arts in therapy. The research was funded by The Foundation for the Advancement of Arts and Letters in Memory of Rudolf Steiner, which Paul formed with some American colleagues for the purpose of researching the arts in therapy.

Beginning of Nordoff and Robbins' Collaboration

At Sunfield Paul began working with groups of children and soon began to see some of them individually. He collaborated with several teachers and classes; one teacher in particular had an intuitive empathy for his work and they

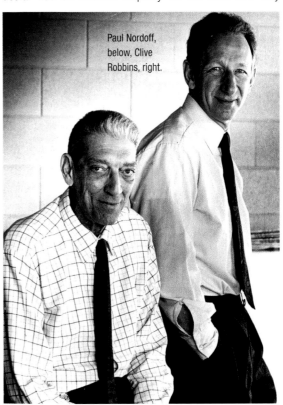

Paul Nordoff, below, Clive Robbins, right.

Johnny

Johnny was an autistic boy with extreme behavioural disturbance and withheld communication, who came to live at Sunfield at about the same time that Paul Nordoff arrived. He was the first child with whom Paul worked individually; initially, Hep Geuter asked Paul to spend half an hour alone with Johnny, simply playing the piano for him and observing his responses. Later in the day, Paul reported his findings at Johnny's case review. He had improvised music in time with Johnny's steps as he walked about the room, and he had alternated between two musical scales – the traditional Eastern pentatonic, with its open, calm quality, and an altered pentatonic that was more dissonant. Intriguingly, this supposedly 'unresponsive' child burst into tears whenever the dissonant music began, and ceased crying when Paul returned to the Eastern pentatonic.

Paul was asked to continue working with Johnny, and saw him three times a week. Johnny gradually relaxed as Paul improvised music attending closely to his moods. The barriers were lowered a little: his attentiveness to Paul increased, their relationship grew, and after seven months, when the programme concluded, Johnny was sleeping better at night and was given a much lighter medication.

quickly developed a special relationship – this was Clive Robbins. Together Paul and Clive developed several musical plays out of folk tales in which the children became profoundly involved in the stories through active musical participation. With the help of Paul's carefully chosen harmonies, appealing melodies and rhythms, the children developed discipline, concentration, self-control and increased social and self-awareness, and for months afterwards they continued to sing and act the songs as they went about their daily life. Paul and Clive also wrote a number of 'play-songs' during that first term, designed to raise the children's awareness of self and surroundings –

songs about the weather, the children's names and clothes and the days of the week, for example.

They began to see children individually as well. Clive's awareness and sensitivity, both musical and personal, made him an ideal co-worker in the room. The children, often placed in front of a snare drum and cymbal, revealed in their responses to Paul's music their sensitivities and capacities, their expressive, receptive and relational abilities. Each child reacted differently to music, and in doing so made a musical *self-portrait* which could be useful for diagnosis and for assessing the child's needs and potentialities. Paul and Clive observed how even subtle developments in the children's abilities that took place in these music sessions, over time, had an impact on their lives in other contexts.

Paul was incredibly rigorous in the consistency of his investigative approach. It was not a hit-and-miss affair; experimental, yes, but with considered application of techniques tried and found to be effective, coupled with intense observational acuity. The legacy of this approach has informed the training of Nordoff-Robbins music therapists to the present day. Clive recognised it at the time as the answer to his prayer for a palpable new way of transforming the lives of the children at Sunfield. The two men spent more time together, in and out of work: at Paul's chalet near a lake they shared music and poetry, and read anthroposophy together. A prolific creative energy was born out of this collaboration and they recognised a kindred spirit in each other.

From January 1960 they also began to make audio recordings of the work. Clive's technical experience (he had previously worked as a theatre lighting technician) enabled him to make high quality recordings, and as a result an archive exists of almost all of Paul and Clive's professional work together – of outstanding importance as a historical testament to their work, as well as being invaluable for the training of music therapists. At the time, however, the tapes were useful primarily for studying the children's musical responses

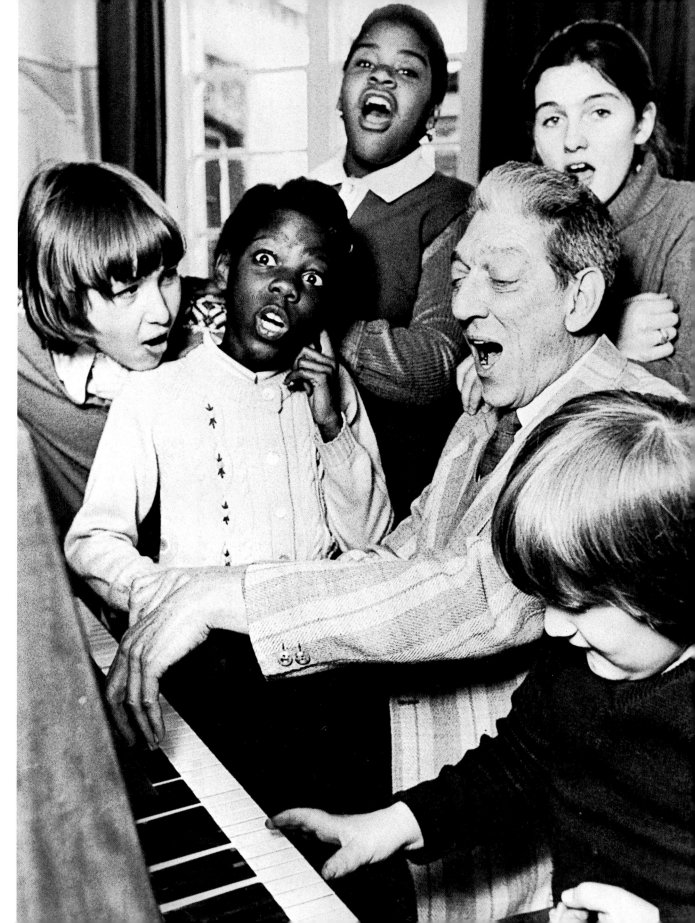

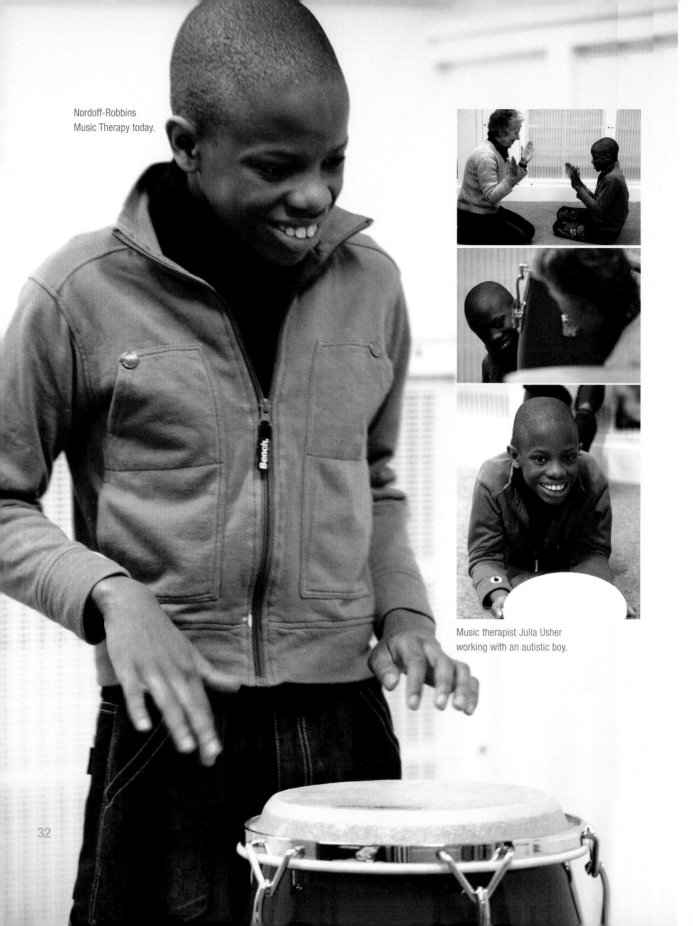

Nordoff-Robbins
Music Therapy today.

Music therapist Julia Usher
working with an autistic boy.

32

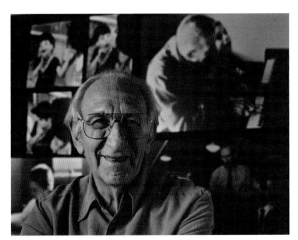

Clive Robbins in 2005.

in greater detail; in time, Paul and Clive also developed sensitive methods of assessing the progress of children over longer periods of time, possible only because of the session recordings.

Beyond Sunfield: development of the work

In the spring of 1960 Paul asked Clive to return with him to America to continue the work. Clive knew that this would mean leaving his wife and children because family life was incompatible with the demands of the work, the intensity and nature of his relationship with Paul and the nomadic existence that they would follow. He made this sacrifice because the grip of the work was so strong.

They left Sunfield in June, and with the continued support of the Foundation for the Advancement of Arts and Letters, undertook a tour of 26 Curative Homes (mainly anthroposophical) across Europe. With all their musical instruments, equipment and tapes, as well as their personal belongings, squeezed into a Ford Consul, they drove through England, Scotland, Sweden, Denmark, Holland, Switzerland and Germany. It was a journey of excitement and discovery, in

Clive Robbins, born 1927

Clive Robbins was born into a baker's family on 23 July 1927 in Handsworth, Birmingham (England), and grew up in a confusion of family relationships caused by the social strategies adopted to hide the shame of illegitimacy in England at that time. It was not until Clive was 17 that he discovered that the woman he had always believed was his older sister was his mother; this lack of a normal maternal relationship created a profound disorientation that left him in search of meaning and purpose in life. Clive developed a lifelong passion for music as a boy. His unhappiness was compounded by the disruption of the Second World War, when he was sent away to foster parents, and listening to classical music (as well as his own piano lessons) brought solace and an 'emotional education', as he later described it.

A serious injury in the RAF at the age of 18 nearly killed Clive, and he survived with partial paralysis of his left hand and arm, which spelled the end of his days as a pianist. His creative talents led him to photography and painting but eventual disillusionment and a succession of dead-end jobs followed.

Returning to his family home in the Midlands in 1950, Clive soon met Mildred, who became his first wife. Mildred began to work as a nurse at an anthroposophical school, Sunfield Children's Homes. When Clive visited he was enchanted by the place, and became a student teacher there in 1954. They lived in the grounds in a small trailer with their two children, Tobias and Jennifer. It was at Sunfield that Clive encountered Paul Nordoff in 1958, and the creative partnership that developed from this meeting set Clive on a lifelong mission. Together they pioneered a music therapy approach that Clive has championed relentlessly: with Nordoff, and (after Nordoff's death) with his second wife, Carol, he has taken it around the world. Clive Robbins is the Founding Director of the Nordoff-Robbins Center for Music Therapy at New York University and lives with his third wife Kaoru, also a music therapist.

which they learned more about approaches to working with mentally disabled children and were able to corroborate the general applicability of the work they had begun. In many homes Paul and Clive gave illustrated presentations, as well as live demonstrations, where children would play with Paul and Clive in front of an audience interested in the work. However, their reception was mixed, with some audiences enthusiastic but others fiercely critical. A number of conventional anthroposophists objected to their use of harshly dissonant and percussive music to express the turbulent lives of disturbed children, and they were viewed as transgressors. This response was bitterly disappointing at first, but it led to the highly successful development of Nordoff-Robbins Music Therapy outside the mainstream tradition of anthroposophy.

Paul and Clive arrived in the USA in late 1960 and spent the next six years establishing a firm basis for their work. They undertook several short-term projects before being awarded a prestigious five-year research grant at the University of Pennsylvania in Philadelphia; this was a Federal grant from the National Institute of Mental Health and the first such award for music therapy. Paul and Clive combined this research with employment as music therapy consultants

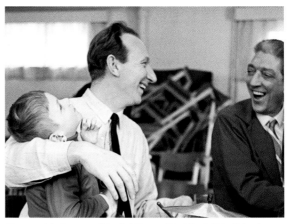

Above and facing page, Clive Robbins and Paul Nordoff, in Finland, express their surprise and delight in a young boy's rhythmic singing.

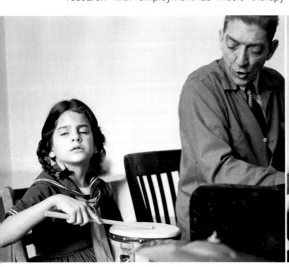
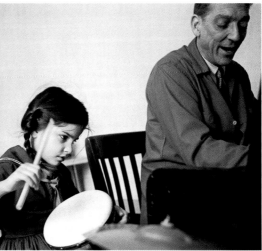
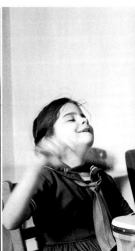

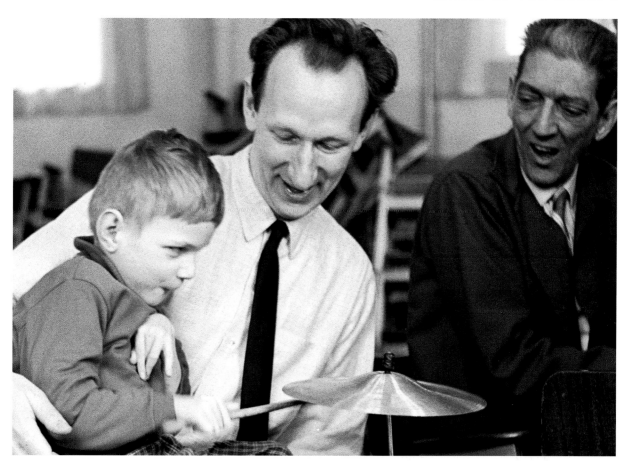

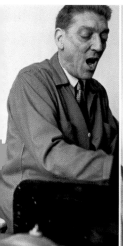
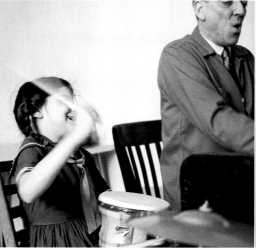
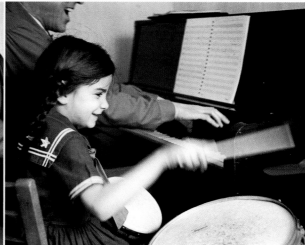

for the School District of Philadelphia. They continued to refine and crystallise the work, always keeping in close contact with Hep Geuter, back at Sunfield, who remained an important mentor. They also began to disseminate their work, publishing their first book, *Music Therapy for Handicapped Children*, 1965, and teaching summer courses at the Crane School of Music at the State University of Potsdam, New York.

In 1967 Paul and Clive were appointed Lecturing Fellows of the American-Scandinavian Foundation. For the next seven years they lived and worked largely in Europe, teach-

ing, writing, giving workshops and continuing the work itself. In Scandinavia they evolved a format for giving short-term, intensive, introductory courses, which led to invitations to teach across Europe. Interest in the work continued to grow: two books appeared in 1971, one of them, *Therapy in Music for Handicapped Children*, a revision of their 1965 book with a foreword by Benjamin Britten; in 1972 a television documentary was made in Norway; and in 1973 they taught a two-month course in Oslo – their longest so far.

Anna

In their book *Creative Music Therapy* (1977) Paul Nordoff and Clive Robbins gave detailed accounts of their work with three children. One of these was a withdrawn 11-year-old girl, Anna, with whom they worked in the unit where she lived. Anna was multiply-disabled, with cerebral palsy, epilepsy and severe visual impairment; she had developed only elementary speech and was isolated from her peers.

In their usual way, Paul sat at the piano while Clive facilitated Anna's physical movements. In her first session Anna made unexpected responses; she beat the drum in time and sang simple musical phrases creatively in dialogue with the therapists, sometimes laughing with pleasure. This was extraordinary because she had had difficulty singing any songs in the classroom as her struggle with verbal pronunciation led her to give up trying. But in this *improvisational* musical situation her slightest sounds were picked up, accompanied and reflected and she was encouraged to develop them.

Anna came twice weekly for music therapy over several months. Her beating of the percussion instruments was brought under firm and conscious control with the assistance of the therapists' directive support; she learned to distinguish the contrasting timbres of drum and cymbal, and to make use of her weaker arm. She learned to locate the instruments in space and derived enormous satisfaction from coordinating her arms to beat them alternately with the biggest, most releasing movements she could make; so although she could not walk through space with her legs, she could experience the satisfaction of marching energetically through powerful music. With her voice she participated in humorous and increasingly complex musical exchanges with the therapists and she learned to sing the words of simple improvised songs. Anna's emphatic exclamations were proof enough, if any were needed, of the immense benefit of this musical experience.

During these weeks Anna carried the effects of her Music Therapy experiences over into other activities: in the classroom she became livelier, and more responsive. After 18 sessions her mother said, 'We are so happy to see Anna so happy and with a certain self-assurance about her.'

Her teachers stated that 'Anna talks a great deal and her speech is becoming more intelligible . . . She picks up new words and puts words together . . . She is well aware of what the other children are doing . . . and she shows a great deal more openness and willingness to accept instruction.'

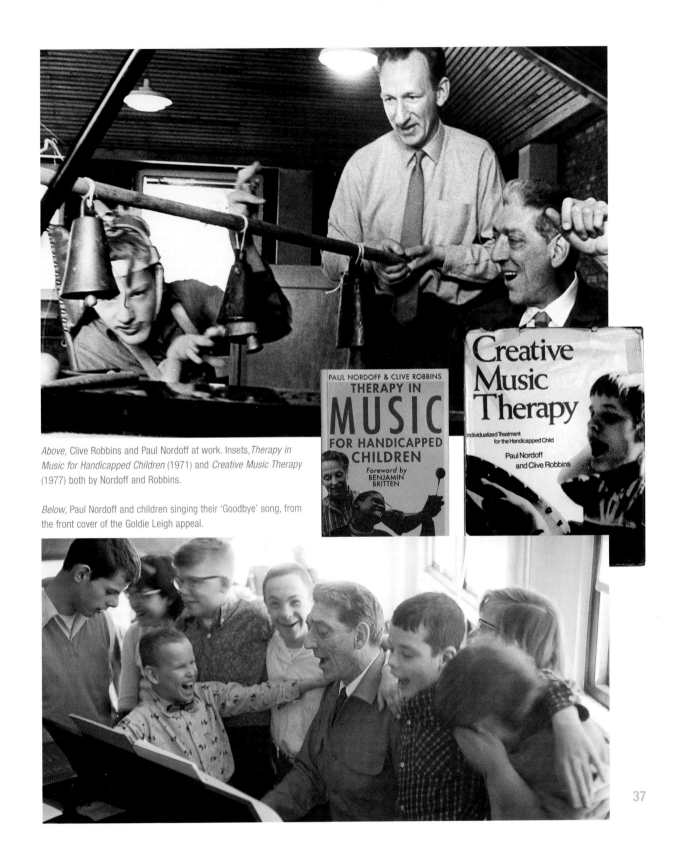

Above, Clive Robbins and Paul Nordoff at work. Insets,*Therapy in Music for Handicapped Children* (1971) and *Creative Music Therapy* (1977) both by Nordoff and Robbins.

Below, Paul Nordoff and children singing their 'Goodbye' song, from the front cover of the Goldie Leigh appeal.

PAUL NORDOFF & CLIVE ROBBINS
THERAPY IN
MUSIC
FOR HANDICAPPED
CHILDREN
Foreword by
BENJAMIN
BRITTEN

Creative
Music
Therapy
Individualized Treatment
for the Handicapped Child
Paul Nordoff
and Clive Robbins

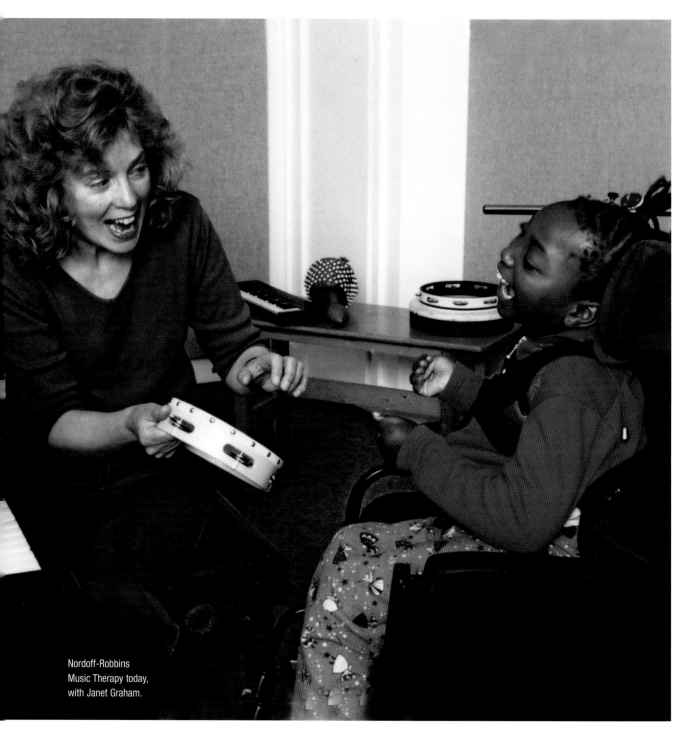

Nordoff-Robbins
Music Therapy today,
with Janet Graham.

Sybil Beresford-Peirse, 1912–2002

Born in Middlesborough on 9 August 1912, Sybil Adelaide Beresford-Peirse was the eldest daughter of a parish priest and granddaughter of the Third Earl of Cawdor. Her childhood was tragically overshadowed by the death of her mother when Sybil was only five years old, an event that undoubtedly had a profound and formative effect on her, perhaps contributing to her tough character and the determination for which she became renowned in later life. She trained in music from an early age, receiving piano lessons from Mabel Lander (a pupil of Leschetizky) and later entering the Royal Academy of Music.

Sybil went on to have a distinguished career in music education and teacher training. Among her many posts, she was Head of Music at The Froebel Demonstration School, Roehampton (1940–55), Head of Music at Offley Training College, Hitchin, Hertfordshire (1947–61) and Head of Music at Sidney Webb College of Education, Westminster (1961–67). She had a passion for encouraging children to express themselves which long pre-dated her discovery of music therapy: piano teaching for her was a dynamic process in which a child's whole being was nurtured, developed and supported.

With the benefit of hindsight, Sybil's interests and passions seem almost destined to bring her into the sphere of work that was becoming known, by the 1960s, as music therapy. Her childhood in a priestly home exposed her to the notion of the Christian life primarily as one of service, crossing boundaries of class and working particularly with the underprivileged. She also inherited her father's considerable gifts of persuasion and talent for raising money (according to one story, whenever one of Reverend Richard Beresford-Peirse's parishioners caught sight of him in the street, it was cheaper for them to hail a taxi and flee than be confronted with their vicar's latest fund-raising effort). Her aristocratic upbringing gave her inside experience and an intimate understanding of social protocol and diplomacy as well as valuable contacts, all of which were to stand her in good stead as she gathered around her a committee of supporters and fund-raisers who were to form the bedrock on which the Nordoff-Robbins charity could grow.

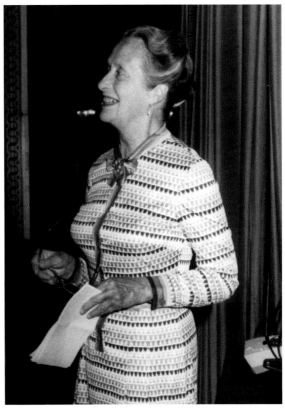

Sybil Beresford-Peirse.

Interest grows in England

By this time, Paul and Clive had already been in touch for several years with a formidable lady named Sybil Beresford-Peirse, who became the seminal figure in the establishment of Nordoff-Robbins Music Therapy in Britain. When Sybil first encountered music therapy she was already in her mid-50s, and it was a mark of her energy and tenacity that she could think of taking up something entirely new and throw herself into it with such zeal.

In 1967 Sybil resigned from her teaching commitments to undertake the first full-time, one-year music therapy training programme in Britain, which took place at the Guildhall School

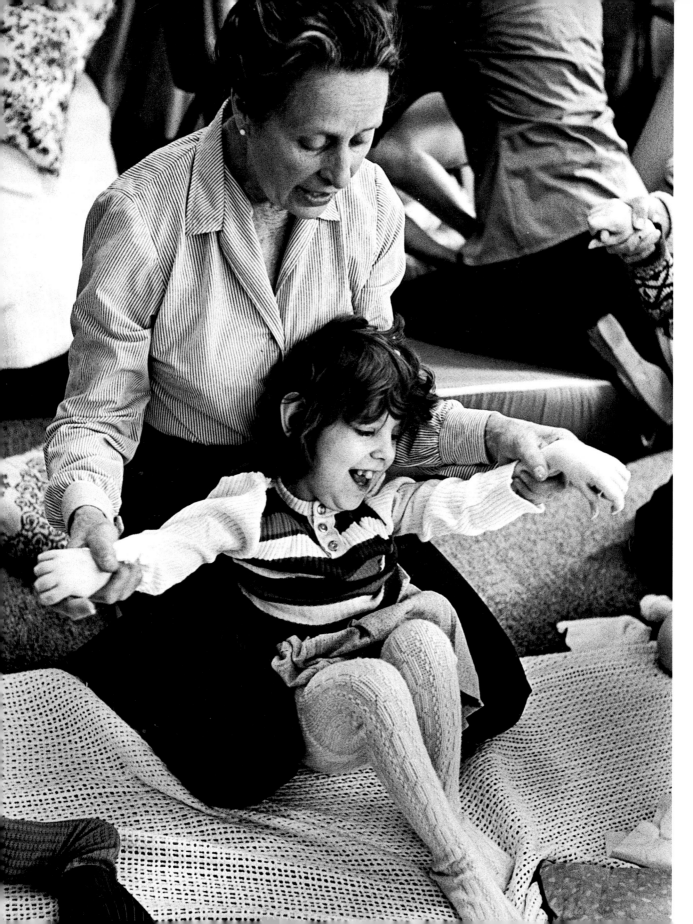

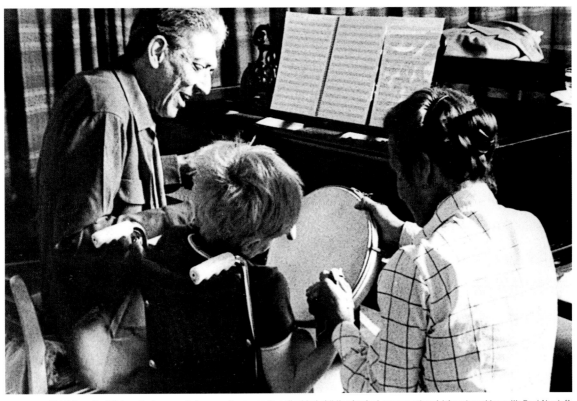

Sybil Beresford-Peirse (facing page) sings as she supports a disabled child's physical movement and (above) working with Paul Nordoff.

of Music and Drama, led by Juliette Alvin (1897–1982), a well-known concert cellist. The course was organised by the Society for Music Therapy and Remedial Music – later the British Society for Music Therapy (BSMT) – which Juliette had formed with colleagues in 1958. The music therapy profession was still in its infancy, and significant though the establishment of the Guildhall programme was, the work was experimental. The notion of musical *co-improvisation* as a basis for music therapy, which was to be the great contribution of Paul Nordoff and Clive Robbins to the field, was largely unknown in Britain. Juliette was aware of their work, however (initially through Herbert Geuter, who had joined the BSMT): in 1963 and 1965 she had invited them to speak at BSMT meetings, and on the 1967/68 training programme she played a tape of

their work, which they had made especially for her. Sybil Beresford-Peirse was one of several students on the Guildhall course who went on to explore the Nordoff-Robbins work further, attracted by the practical and systematic approach they had developed. Inspired by their first book, *Music Therapy for Handicapped Children*, which she read in one sitting, Sybil resolved to go and meet Nordoff and Robbins and bring their work to Britain.

She met Paul and Clive in 1968 in Philadelphia where she heard them lecture about their work with autistic children and afterwards declared her commitment to their approach. The two men were naturally enthusiastic, and Sybil returned home enthused. She began to set up a music therapy clinical practice for herself, initially at three London schools with facilities for chil-

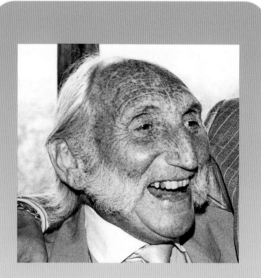

Dr David Morris, FRCP, MRCS, DCH
1915–89

A colourful, dapper figure, who always sported a rose in his buttonhole, Dr David Morris became a consultant paediatrician at Goldie Leigh Hospital in 1960. At a time when educational provision for such children was still extremely poor, Morris was among those visionaries who led the way in creating a better present and future for them, and was much loved by the children in his care. He was present at the gathering in Sybil's home in September 1970, when Paul and Clive presented their work to a group of interested professionals, and he recognised its potential for enabling disabled children to develop to their optimum and lead more significant lives. He immediately introduced it at Goldie Leigh, and remained a wholehearted supporter for the rest of his life. For Sybil and her colleagues it was a great coup to win the professional support of such an eminent paediatrician. David Morris was to play an active role in the affairs of Nordoff-Robbins Music Therapy until his death, teaching on the training programme and serving for many years as Chairman of the Board of Governors. He was a wise advisor to whom Sybil turned frequently.

dren with special education needs. Sybil incorporated some of the techniques from the Nordoff-Robbins work, making use of and adapting some of the Nordoff-Robbins compositions. She also maintained frequent, often voluminous correspondence with Paul and Clive, and joined the growing international circle of interested practitioners for whom Paul and Clive were circulating a library of clinical studies on tape. Sybil was also asked to try out a set of rating scales that Paul and Clive were developing to evaluate children's progress in music therapy. This valuable clinical tool offered concrete, systematic and practical goals, and Sybil was thrilled with it; as Clive later recalled: 'it was as if we had sent her the keys to the kingdom.'

Sybil arranged for Paul and Clive to lecture in London, organising two weekend presentations in 1970 at her home in Holland Park. These were the first of many introductory presentations and courses that Sybil would organise, though already she had set her sights much higher. The vision of a one-year training programme, taught by Paul and Clive, was an ambitious conception, but Sybil and her vision, determination, administrative acumen and personal contacts proved equal to the challenge.

Establishing a centre for music therapy

At the invitation of Dr David Morris, one of Sybil's colleagues, Julienne Cartwright (a fellow student of Sybil on the first Guildhall course) began music therapy work at Goldie Leigh Hospital in 1970. Like Sybil, Julienne had become enthused by Nordoff and Robbins' work and was applying their approach. However, Julienne only worked at Goldie Leigh for a year (she was later a key figure in the establishment of Nordoff-Robbins Music Therapy in Scotland), and Sybil was invited to continue the work in 1971, assisted by Jenny Bates, who had also trained on the Guildhall programme. Like Nordoff and Robbins, they considered individual therapy to be the very core of the work through which the most withdrawn or dis-

Goldie Leigh Hospital

Goldie Leigh Children's Cottage Homes opened in 1902 as an orphanage for up to 300 children, east of the City of London (near Abbey Wood). The attractive rural setting and home-like design of the 11 buildings represented a marked ideological and political shift of values from the austere and barren workhouses of Victorian times. However, by 1914 the work of social reformers, such as Thomas J. Barnardo, had led to widespread alternative provision for orphans and deserted children, and Goldie Leigh became a hospital for children suffering from tuberculosis and, later, diseases of the skin and scalp, notably eczema and ringworm.

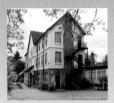

The discovery of penicillin in 1928 heralded a new era of anti-biotic treatment, which became widely available in the late 1940s and the need for a large hospital like Goldie Leigh declined. In 1960 Goldie Leigh began providing residential care for up to 120 children with mental and physical disabilities, from south east England. Further alterations were made over the next decade to accommodate more severely disabled children, although the remaining skin units were not finally closed until 1976.

turbed child could be reached. Group work offered expanded opportunities for the children to experiment with and further develop their new-found social and communicative skills, enabling them to experience the satisfaction of attainment with their peers. Another form of group work was also developed for the most physically and mentally impaired children. With the assistance of Sheila Tyler, the head physiotherapist, and her colleagues, sessions were established on one of the wards, in which music was provided to support the gentle facilitation of movement and easing of physical stiffness. Simple and memorable songs, often including the names of the children, encouraged their awareness and participation. The results were often remarkable, with music lighting up the faces of children who responded to nothing else.

Meanwhile, as she developed as a clinician, Sybil was nourished by Paul and Clive's many letters and their visits. She sometimes sent them recordings of her work on which they commented in detail. When they came to London to give presentations she was able to share her work with them and

they visited some of her clinical sites.

The presentations given by Nordoff and Robbins in London were often at Goldie Leigh. Live demonstrations, with children, were conducted for the audience, followed by in-depth discussion. Rachel Verney vividly recaptured the atmosphere of one such lecture-demonstration in 1972, her first encounter with the work:

> I was sitting in this huge, echoey hall fairly near the back. Right down at the front there was this piano and this man sitting at it, and a very large adolescent boy was brought in and was banging around on this drum. There was another man sort of dancing around him. There was a lot of energy, and it was all wild and chaotic. It didn't make any sense to me at all, except that the energy was very clear, particularly from the man (Paul Nordoff) at the piano.

Anybody who has heard any of the tapes of Nordoff and

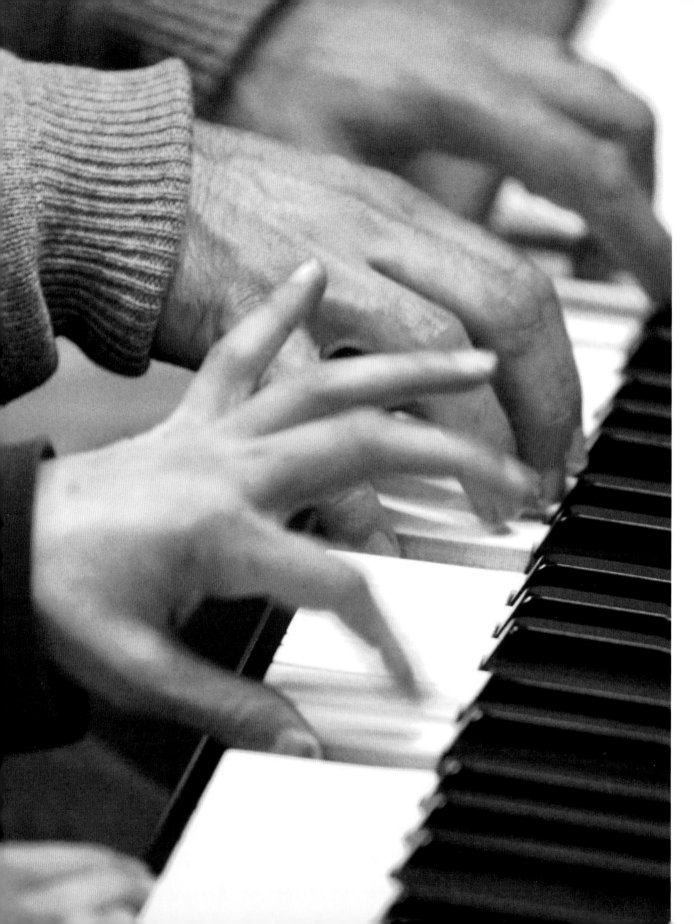

Robbins' work will have some idea of that spellbinding life and energy which they offered their clients in the drama of musical experience.

The Nordoff-Robbins Project Committee and emergent training programme

In October 1971 Sybil Beresford-Peirse gathered together a committee of professionals from the musical and medical professions, chaired by Dr Morris. Her aim was the establishment of a one-year, full-time training programme at Goldie Leigh, for which at least £12,000 would need to be raised. On 7 March 1972 the committee met with representatives of the Music Therapy Charity, an Oxford-based organisation that had been formed in 1968 to raise funds in aid of music therapy. Sybil knew one of the governors of this charity, Mary, Countess of Bradford (1918–86), as they were old school friends. Paul and Clive were also present. The Music Therapy Charity, under its Chairman, Lady Alexandra Trevor-Roper (1907–97), agreed to work with Sybil's committee (the Nordoff-Robbins Project Committee), with the intention of setting up a training programme at Goldie Leigh and a permanent centre for the work.

By degrees, the necessary funds were accrued. Events were organised, such as a celebrity fashion show at Weston Park in Shropshire, the home of Lady Bradford, which brought in £6,000. Meanwhile, there was preparation work to be done at Goldie Leigh. The training programme would need space: the pioneers at Goldie Leigh had had to work wherever they could find privacy and a piano (some individual sessions took place in the laundry room cupboard!). With the support of the hospital manager, Mr Lash, himself a keen musician, an old brick outhouse was converted to create a sizeable workroom that functioned both as lecture room and therapy room with an observation booth. A small office and the students' common room were located in a neighbouring building.

With Paul and Clive, Sybil planned and organised the training programme. Throughout much of 1972 and 1973, Paul and Clive were hard at work on their book, *Creative Music Therapy*. Though it was not to be published until 1977, they wanted to have the manuscript ready for the course at Goldie Leigh as a central focus for the teaching material. Slowly the book progressed, with Sybil's demands for the latest chapter often keeping them on schedule.

At the same time, the BBC made a small documentary about the music therapy work at Goldie Leigh. As a result of this programme, a good lady, aged 85, presented them with a splendid Bechstein grand piano. Sybil finally got the course approved by the government Department of Education and Science and she assembled a group of 13 students to undertake it, through a formal interview process. Everything was ready by January 1974 when the training programme began.

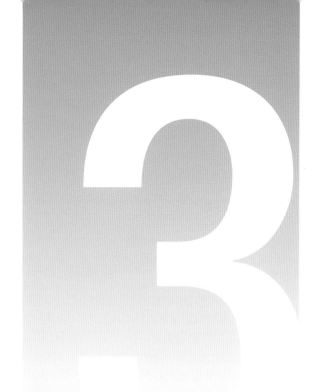

They were an incredible partnership
. . . I don't know how they did it. It
was like a duet . . . utterly riveting.

Jane Gibson

Secure Foundations

The first training programme at Goldie Leigh

The first Nordoff-Robbins programme was an acclaimed achievement and set a blueprint for training. Entitled the Nordoff-Robbins Preliminary Training Course in Music Therapy, it ran for six months at Goldie Leigh Hospital. Fifteen students from five countries followed the programme which was taught mainly by Paul and Clive and administered by Sybil Beresford-Peirse who also participated as a student. While the programme has obviously evolved over the succeeding 30 years, it has retained the basic fundamental structure established in 1974.

The heart of the course involved the acquisition of specific music improvisation skills, together with an understanding of, and competence in, their clinical application. Paul Nordoff gave two inspirational sets of interactive and musically illustrated lectures (entitled 'Talks on Music' and 'Instructions in Improvisation') about the language, construction and emotional impact of music; examining the great composers, he dissected their music into basic elements, including scales and tonalities, tonal direction, melodic and harmonic construction, intervals, triads and inversions, sevenths, tension and resolution, and musical 'archetypes'. The students were taught to understand, in precise and practical detail, how music engages people. The lectures were complemented by Paul and Clive's teaching, comprising the theory of the approach, case studies, clinical techniques, applications and evaluation scales. One student, Jane Worthington (later Gibson), who went on to teach musical resources to students for many years, recalled her experience of this:

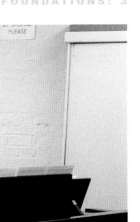

Jane Gibson facilitates a physically disabled child, supported by Robin Howat at the piano.

They were an incredible partnership when they shared their teachings. One would say a sentence and then the other would say something. I don't know how they did it, it was incredible. It was like a duet. They would come in with different aspects and angles and it was very invigorating and utterly riveting.

From the observation booth, the students watched Paul and Clive working in individual sessions with children, and as the students became more experienced they began to work with children themselves, supervised by Paul and Clive. A variety of different conditions and needs were presented, and the students not only observed each other's work from the booth, but also took turns in providing a running commentary of sessions on tape. Supporting lectures were provided by Dr David Morris, who gave a medical background to disability and disease, and Dr Mel Marshak, who offered a psychotherapeutic perspective on the work and on child development.

Paul Nordoff was a man with a powerful and commanding presence, and the students were both awed and inspired by him. Furthermore, he was not in good health, and there was some urgency in his desire to communicate and share the depths of his work so that others would be able to continue it. He tolerated nothing less than total commitment, and his expectations of the students were high. One can imagine the electric atmosphere, and the intimidating task for students of going out and performing in front of their tutors and peers.

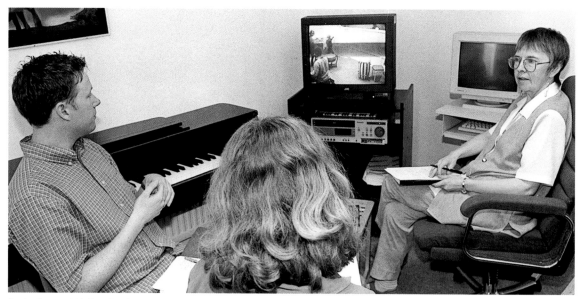

Sandra Brown, right, Year One Coordinator and Clinical Supervisor, analysing video recordings of students' training sessions during supervision.

The 15 students all graduated successfully in July 1974, and a number of them went on to make major contributions to the development of both Nordoff-Robbins Music Therapy and the wider profession of music therapy in the UK and elsewhere.

Paul and Clive's separation

A whole year was to pass before a second training programme could run, and there were two major reasons for this; one was a general shortage of funds and the other was a turbulent and protracted separation between Paul and Clive through 1974, which left the future unclear. This was something that had been brewing for some time, as Clive later remembered:

> By the end of 1973 we were both outgrowing our relationship . . . I was also feeling that what I did was

imprisoning him . . . We both individually had to move beyond the confines of this very strong team we had built up. My thinking-life, my feeling-life, even the way I thought about anthroposophy, was moving in a different direction to Paul's.

The Goldie Leigh training was a fantastic culmination of the years of Paul and Clive's devotion to the work; an achievement they had long hoped for and dreamed of. In Clive's words, it was 'the secure foundation we had always been seeking.' Their parting represented both an end and a new beginning, inevitable and important. Herbert Geuter, who had mentored them for 15 years, continued to support them both, and made it clear that he felt that the end of their teamwork would make greater things possible. Paul returned to Philadelphia where he began treatment for prostate cancer; the early diagnosis was for a full recovery, but time would reveal it as a lengthy, terminal illness.

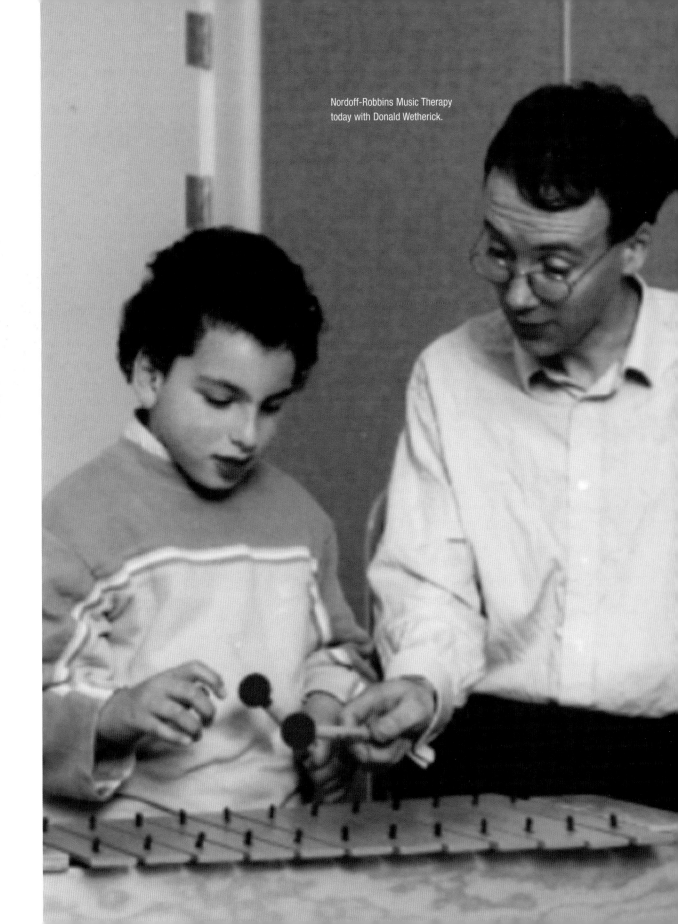

Nordoff-Robbins Music Therapy
today with Donald Wetherick.

EVERY NOTE COUNTS: THE STORY OF NORDOFF-ROBBINS MUSIC THERAPY

As the dust settled, everyone realised that Paul and Clive's personal difficulties could not be allowed to prevent the work from continuing and expanding, and a second programme was planned in which Paul and Clive would teach separately. In the initial aftermath of the separation, Sybil sided heavily with Paul and renamed the Goldie Leigh department the Nordoff Music Therapy Centre, removing Clive's name. Fortunately, the omission would not be a permanent one, since Clive's contribution to the work was no less essential than Paul's, but it remained until after Paul's death in 1977. It was shortly after this that Sybil was persuaded that Clive's name should be reinstated, though her relationship with him remained rocky for some time.

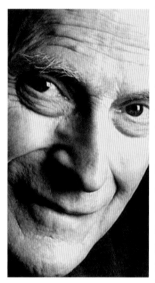

Yehudi Menuhin wrote, 'I can think of no more exciting and promising effort . . .'

The Service of Dedication at Westminster Abbey

The Music Therapy Charity was working hard to interest the classical music establishment in the Nordoff-Robbins work, and to this end Lady Alexandra Trevor-Roper and Lady Bradford decided to organise a grand service of dedication for the Music Therapy Charity in Westminster Abbey. With an invited guest list of hundreds, from royalty to business executives, this significant event took place in June 1975, and featured a number of celebrities, including Yehudi Menuhin, who performed on the violin, and Richard Baker and Dame Anna Neagle, who read lessons. Both Paul and Clive were present.

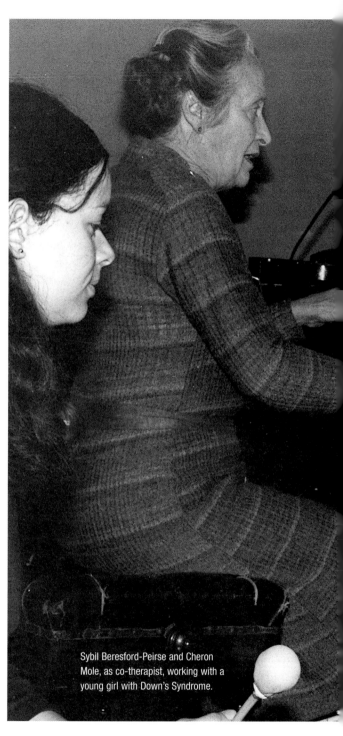

Sybil Beresford-Peirse and Cheron Mole, as co-therapist, working with a young girl with Down's Syndrome.

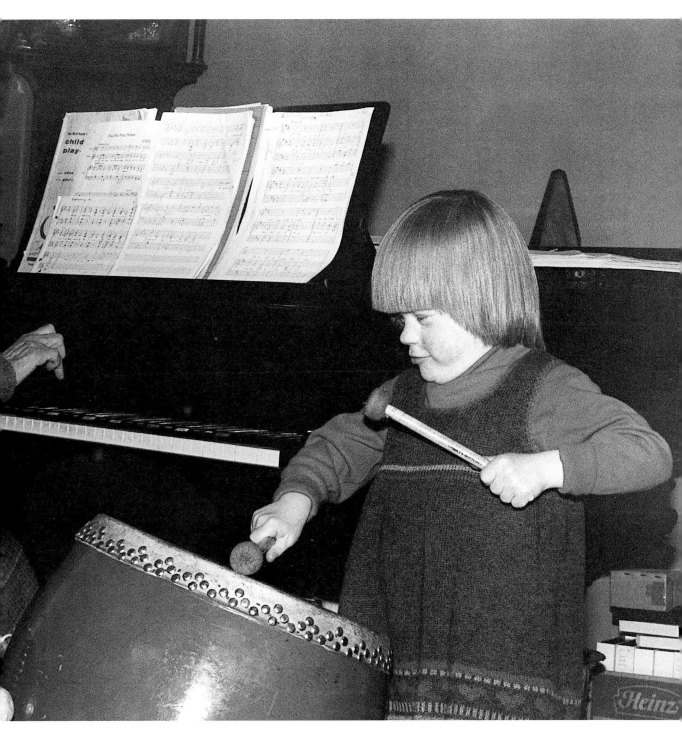

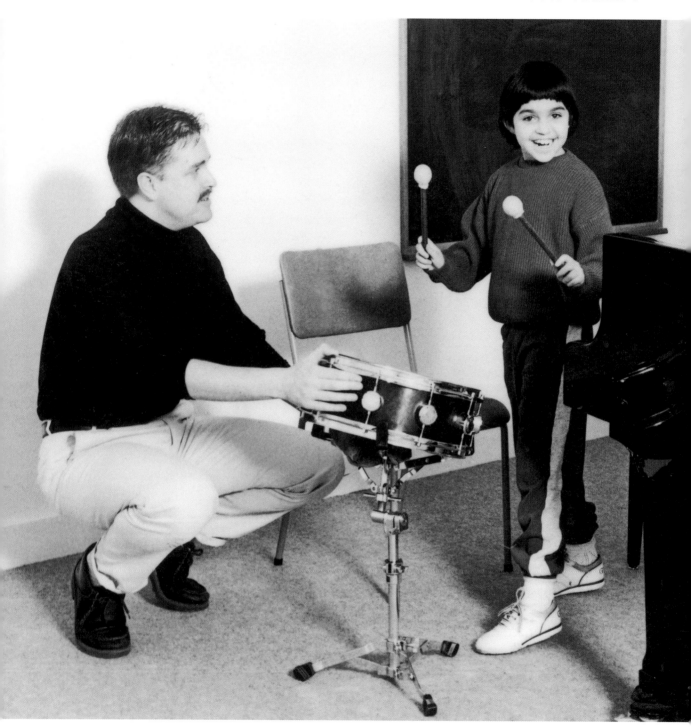

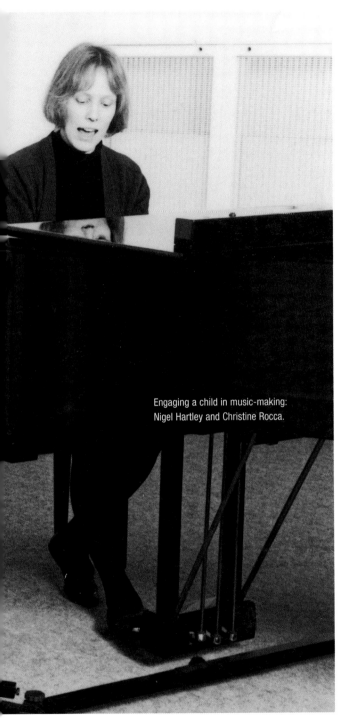

Engaging a child in music-making:
Nigel Hartley and Christine Rocca.

The concert enthralled many; none more so than Nancy Jarratt, UK Director of Moët & Chandon champagne. She immediately wrote to Lady Bradford to ask if there was anything she could do to help. That letter marked the beginning of over 30 years of tireless, invaluable work for Nordoff-Robbins, and Nancy continues to support the charity today as a member of the Board of Governors and Fund-Raising Committee.

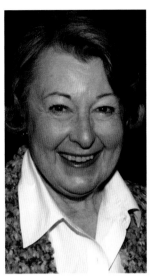

Nancy Jarratt

The Westminster Abbey concert proved that classical musicians were supportive of the cause. This and other events provided useful publicity for Nordoff-Robbins, but the classical music industry simply did not generate enough money to be able to secure the continuation of the work and training programme.

The second training programme

A year after the first programme finished, enough money had been scraped together for it to run again. Meanwhile, the department at Goldie Leigh had expanded, employing three of the new graduates, Jean Eisler, Jane Gibson and Jane Healey. Sybil also acquired a second-hand Portakabin that greatly increased the available space.

The second training ran for the full academic year 1975/76. Sybil held it together even more comprehensively than she had the first year. With Paul and Clive teaching separately, it was down to her to plan the structure and oversee the programme as a whole. It was an invaluable experience for her because she could still consult Paul, but the next time she would be faced with the unenviable role of transmitting his teaching herself. Clive had by now remarried and was living in the USA; his new American wife, Carol, an ardent student of Paul Nordoff and gifted improviser, was also a music therapist, and they were establishing work together at the New York State School for the Deaf. Clive responded magnanimously to the removal of his name at Goldie Leigh, and he and Carol came over twice during the course to work with students. Once again, the absolute core musical training came from Paul, who planned his seminars about music and improvisation resources in a similar way to the previous year. After sessions the students would sit with Paul, who would go through the recording of the session in minute detail. This was the very core of his knowledge, brilliance and insight – his understanding of how people can be called to life through music. The other significant addition to the tutorial team was Alfred Nieman (1913–97), composition teacher at the

Guildhall School of Music and Drama, who taught the students keyboard improvisation. He would remain a valued member of staff throughout the development of the Nordoff-Robbins programme, until his retirement in 1991.

The Junior Fund-Raising Committee

By the summer of 1976, as the completion of the second course approached the financial situation became desperate. Sybil had accrued a £6,000 overdraft and it seemed a miracle was needed.

Mary Bradford was passionate about the cause and was working on a new plan. Towards the end of 1975 she had approached a talented young concert promoter in the rock music industry, who also happened to be the son of her GP back in Shropshire. Andrew Miller was only in his 20s, but had already made a name for himself and was mixing with many of the big names in rock 'n' roll. He was fascinated to hear about

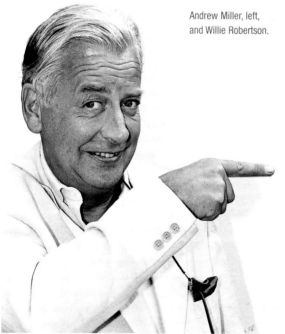

Andrew Miller, left, and Willie Robertson.

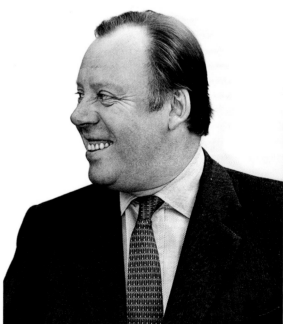

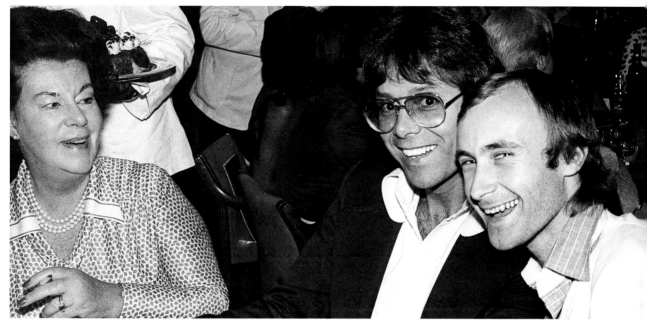

Left to right, Lady Bradford, Cliff Richard and Phil Collins
at an early fund-raising event.

the idea of music as therapy, and Mary spared him none of the details of the critical financial circumstances facing the establishment at Goldie Leigh. Although at this time there were big charities in show business, such as the Variety Club, none were supported by the rock music industry specifically, and Andrew felt this void had potential. He was summoned to a meeting in Wimpole Street with some of the Music Therapy Charity ladies, as well as David Morris and Nancy Jarratt. Andrew recalled this rather intimidating experience:

> I remember being very embarrassed because I was there with very long hair and a velvet suit, the trendy things that one wore in those days . . . and they sort of grilled me and said, 'What can you do?' They made it absolutely clear that they were desperate for money, and they were so desperate that the whole thing was about to collapse unless they had an immediate injection of funds. I made

it clear that the only way that I could possibly help would be by forming a fund-raising committee within the contemporary music industry and reporting back to them with ways in which we thought we could help them as a collective body. So they gave me authority that evening to do that.

Andrew's sphere of activity was a world away from the aristocratic circles of the Oxford-based Music Therapy Charity, and he knew that he would need to establish a separate operation. The committee that he put together over the next few weeks became known as the Junior Fund-Raising Committee (of the Music Therapy Charity), and was the embryonic form of what would eventually become the Nordoff-Robbins Music Therapy Charity. Andrew's friend, Willie Robertson, an insurance broker in the music industry, was first on board, and together they made some grand plans: 'I said to him, "I'll tell

A 'Damascene' Conversion

Like others who were becoming involved with the Junior Fund-Raising Committee, rock band manager Sam Alder, *right,* went to Goldie Leigh one day to see for himself what their efforts were in aid of. He was accompanied by Steve O'Rourke, manager of Pink Floyd, and they were taken inside the music therapy room to watch a session from the observation booth. Sam remembers:

It was the first time I saw Sybil Beresford-Peirse in action. An unfortunate child was brought in who was doing a repetitive rocking movement that was just going on and on and on. I actually went with great apprehension because as a non-medical person who is rarely ill I had the illogical fear of mental illness that lots of people have who find it difficult to face that sort of thing . . . These crashing chords came out of the piano, and I was sitting there thinking, This is terrifying! Is this what music therapy is about, these crashing chords and the child's head rocking? And then I suddenly realised that the chords and the head movements were together. And then the chords slowed down, and the head movements slowed down with them and stopped, and I suddenly realised the nurse next to me was in tears.

From that day Sam Alder was totally committed to the cause, supporting the charity for over 30 years and playing a central role in its corporate development. From 1997 to 2007 he acted as Chairman of the Board of Governors, and was a wise advisor to successive Directors of the charity.

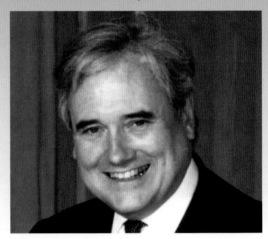

you what, Willie. Let's crack open another bottle of wine and I'm going to make myself Chairman and I want you to be my Vice-Chairman." And I think after our third bottle of wine we had settled that!'

A broad mix of people in the business was needed to handle various facets of the enterprise – fund-raising, accounting and public profiling. City financiers Peter Robertson (Willie's brother) and Neil Edmonstone were persuaded to join the team, and Nancy Jarratt was enlisted as Secretary, bringing invaluable skills in fund-raising and marketing. Other early additions included Sam Alder, then manager of Roxy Music, who became Treasurer, Dave Dee, a record company executive and former pop star, Dee Dee Wilde, a dancer with Pan's People, and the BBC's Michael Appleton, producer of *The Old Grey Whistle Test.* Nancy Jarratt kindly offered the newly formed committee the boardroom at Moët & Chandon for their first meeting, where remarkably they carried on meeting for the next 15 years!

The First Silver Clef Lunch

The rock music industry obviously generated an enormous amount of money, but the crucial question was how this wealth could be tapped. Andrew recalled members of the committee racking their brains:

The committee convened and I did the best I could to explain clinically what we were trying to do . . . I said,

'We need to pay off the overdraft to keep Clive and Paul's work going, so we need £6,000.' I explained that to the committee and then we all sat around and looked at each other after copious amounts of Nancy's champagne and thought, 'What are we going to do?' We had to start getting serious, so we all said that we have to invent an award.

It was a great idea to try to establish a music industry award as a focus for the fund-raising. It would need careful planning for the industry to take it seriously, and Andrew had encountered some scepticism while putting the committee together. They would hold a gourmet lunch in the West End, during which an award would be presented for outstanding contribution to music. The award would need a catchy name, and Andrew remembers it was Dee Dee Wilde who came up with the name Silver Clef.

A date was set for 29 June 1976, just six weeks away, and a large hotel, Park Lane's Inn On The Park, was booked. The pressure was on, and Nancy Jarratt's experience of running publicity events was invaluable. Twiggy, a well-known, popular figure in the business, was asked to present the

Left to right, Willie Robertson, Vice-Chairman, Andrew Miller, Chairman and Sam Alder, Treasurer of the Junior Fund-Raising Committee, 1978.

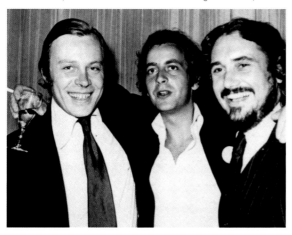

award, which was offered to The Who, one of the biggest bands in 1976 with a decade of successful hits to its name. Both graciously accepted, really as a favour to those organising it, since nobody knew anything about music therapy, nor anticipated the prestige that the award would develop in the ensuing years. To raise awareness about the cause, Paul Nordoff, who was by now a very sick man, was invited to speak because the committee knew it was the power of the work itself that would reach people more than anything else. The 400 people who attended were moved by Paul's brilliant speech. The reputation established at that first Lunch has been the basis for its success ever since. A tremendous £12,000 was raised that day – double what the committee set out to achieve. Each year that success has been repeated and the Silver Clef Award has become one of the most prestigious awards within the contemporary music industry, presented annually to an artist or group for outstanding contribution to music.

Paul Nordoff's death

The Silver Clef Lunch in 1976 secured the immediate future of the Nordoff-Robbins training programme. Nevertheless, there was no training during the 1976/77 academic year, partly because the money came in too late, but also because Paul Nordoff was dying and Sybil could not at this point conceive of running a programme without him.

Paul lived through the final months of his illness in Germany at Herdecke Hospital, dying there on 18 January 1977, aged 67. He was nursed by the anthroposophical principles by which he had lived and worked for so much of his life. Many of his former colleagues and pupils visited him during this time, including Clive Robbins after some two years of occasional contact only; this proved a favourable encounter, in which Paul agreed to add a codicil to his will, assigning the effects of their work – the session tapes, photos, notes and written materials

– to Clive. This final meeting was immensely important for Clive as, resulting from his and Carol's summer courses at New York University, he was being approached regarding the viability of establishing a Nordoff-Robbins Center in New York City attached to the University. Paul was immediately enthused by this, and agreed that their names should appear together in the title of the Center. Hence, his agreement to the codicil brought not only personal resolution to their relationship, but also established Clive's authority to secure the future of their work in the USA. Later, when Paul's wishes became known, Clive's name was restored to the London Centre.

Paul's death, however, was a critical and stressful event for Sybil. She had complete conviction in the work and undoubtedly had the administrative skills required, but she faced a tough challenge. The ensuing years would often be difficult and uncertain, and she bore the impact of that perhaps more than anyone. Yet Sybil's achievements were remarkable and she sustained the training programme with incredible single-mindedness. She and all those left behind owed it to Paul to ensure that the legacy of his creative vision would be sustained and developed fruitfully.

Roehampton

In the aftermath of Paul's death, Sybil began to plan a third programme. The second Silver Clef Lunch was held on 30 June 1977 in the presence of HRH The Duchess of Gloucester, repeating and augmenting the huge success of the first year: this time it took place at the Café Royale, with the award presented to Cliff Richard and the Shadows (the following year it was at the Inter-Continental Hotel near Hyde Park Corner, where it continued to be held for the next 29 years). With this fantastic support, the team could begin to plan with confidence, and the third training programme began in September 1977. Thanks to Clive, Paul Nordoff's teaching on the first Goldie Leigh programme in 1974 had

been recorded in full, and Sybil used these tapes as the basis of the course structure. Robin Howat trained that year and remembered how Sybil taught:

> She would play Paul talking and asking a question, and then she'd switch the tape off and we would do what the students had done in 1974 which was to go up to the piano and practice the exercises Paul set. Then the talk would carry on; you wouldn't hear the original students playing – we were the substitutes!

Sybil continued to teach like this throughout her years as Head of Training – to the increasing discontent of students, who felt that something of the immediacy of Paul's dynamic vision was lost by being 'frozen' on the tapes. But in 1977 the recordings were of crucial importance because they enabled Sybil to impart Paul's teaching and keep the programme going.* Clive and Carol also came over to teach together, as they had the previous year.

From this point, the full-time, one-year programme was an annual fixture; however, it was not to continue at Goldie Leigh. Sybil wanted the programme to gain credibility in the

Mercédès Pavlicevic, right, in training at Roehampton with Clive and Carol Robbins, 1981.

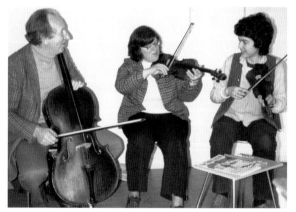

* The tapes were later transcribed and edited by Clive and Carol Robbins, and published in 1998 (see bibliography).

Eleanor

Eleanor was a young woman suffering severe depression, who came to music therapy at her counsellor's suggestion. She had found it difficult to engage in counselling: words just did not seem to come naturally. The counsellor remarked that she seemed frightened to use her voice at all.

In the music therapy room Eleanor found it difficult to make eye contact. She did not seem to know what she wanted to do, so the therapist guided her with some suggestions. Eleanor's playing was hesitant and compliant, and there was no sense of liveliness or spirit. The therapist introduced her to all the instruments in the room and asked her whether she would like to choose one. After some thought, she picked a small, plastic child's recorder and began to play.

Eleanor blew – and blew – and blew. She was not interested in remembering the fingerings. The first sounds were weak, almost inaudible, but as the music therapist improvised at the piano, matching and supporting her, they gradually became stronger and stronger. Eleanor began to vary her breathing to change the sound of the recorder, resulting in a pulsating breathing/sighing/screaming effect. The power of her music was overwhelming, and after 20 minutes it could be sustained no longer. Eleanor and her therapist sat in silence. She was crying.

In subsequent sessions Eleanor began with the recorder before moving on to other instruments. The first week she and her therapist had barely spoken, but slowly she began to talk about herself between their improvisations. Through exploring sounds on the recorder and experiencing the therapist's musical support, however she played, Eleanor found her voice: the unspeakable became speakable. After a few months of music therapy, Eleanor was able to return to counselling.

professional world, which would lead to better job prospects for music therapists, and she also sought official status to help students obtain grants to fund their studies. Furthermore, she aspired to a more spacious venue. Sybil turned to Southlands College of Education – part of Roehampton Institute of Higher Education in south London, where she had professional connections dating back many years – to see whether an amalgamation would be possible. The music department there, under Dr Desmond Sargeant, welcomed the idea and plans were initiated for the establishment of a music therapy unit and the incorporation of the Nordoff-Robbins training programme.

A room was soundproofed and equipped for therapy and observation, and the fourth Nordoff-Robbins training programme began there in September 1978. The new arrangement worked well as the students had access to all the student facilities, and the teaching areas were much better. In other respects, the course remained largely similar to the previous year, but now had the advantage of being a Roehampton-certified diploma course.

Meanwhile, at Goldie Leigh, the work continued to operate for a further 12 years under Jean Eisler's energetic leadership. In the mid-1980s institutional changes at Goldie Leigh led to the relocation of the music therapy department to Wensley Close in Eltham, SE9, where it was incorporated into the new, purpose-built Assessment Centre for early intervention, which exists today under the aegis of Greenwich Healthcare NHS Trust. Music therapy has flourished consistently there, under the leadership first of Julie Allis and then of Sarah Hadley. Today it forms the largest NHS music therapy department in the UK, employing 13 therapists, representing the full spectrum of music therapy training backgrounds.

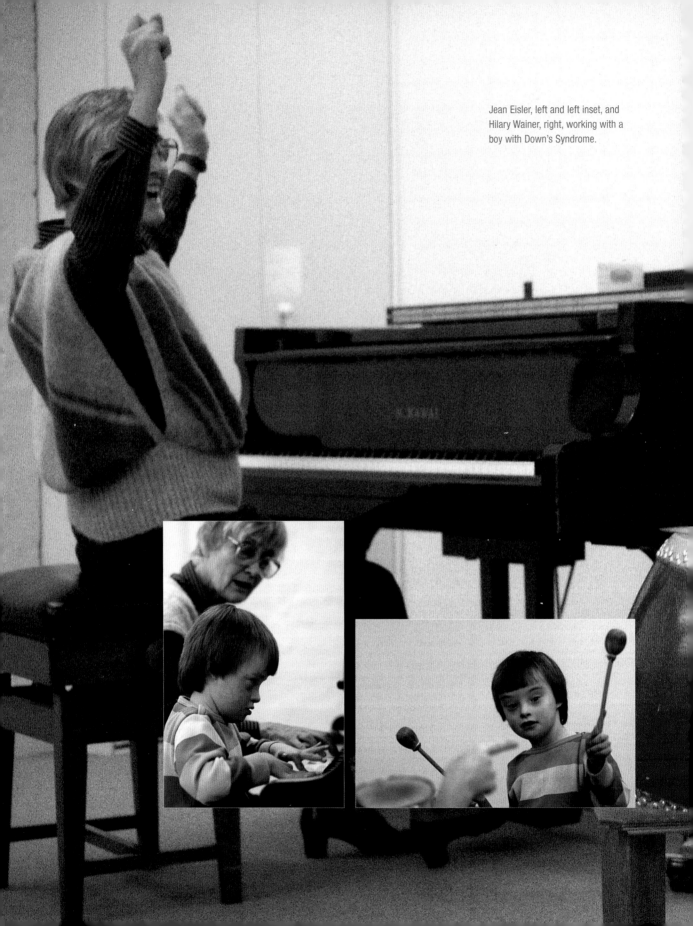

Jean Eisler, left and left inset, and Hilary Wainer, right, working with a boy with Down's Syndrome.

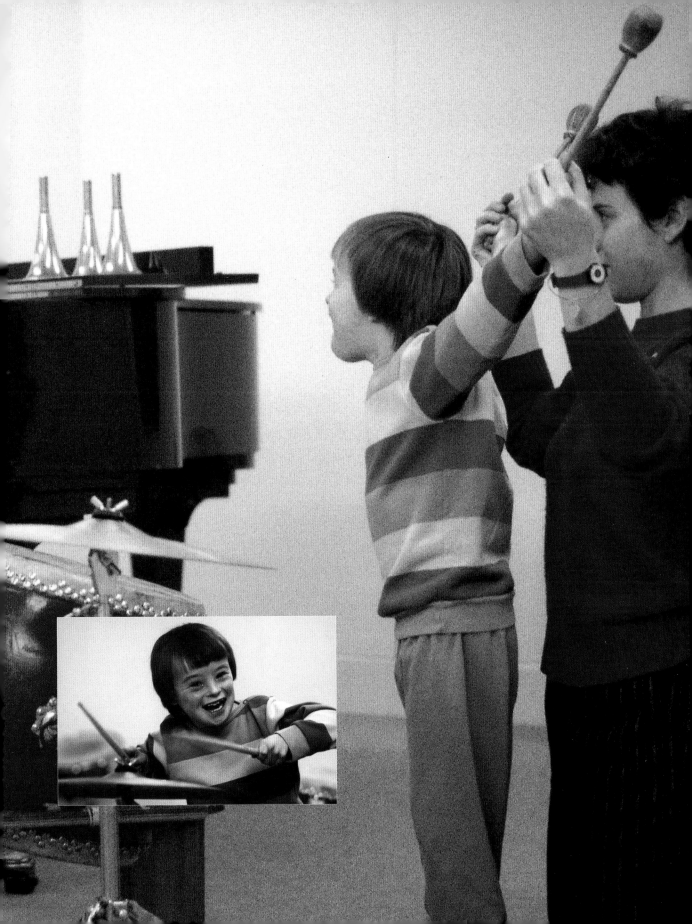

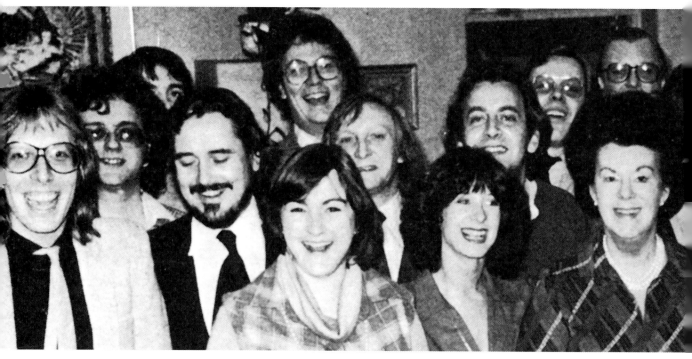

Junior Fund-Raising Committee, 1978:

Left to right, Tony Brainsby, *unknown*, Tony Appleton (BBC), Sam Alder (Treasurer), Benita Haddon, Tony Roberts, Tony Burfield, Dee Dee Wilde, Andrew Miller (Chairman), Willie Robertson (Vice-Chairman), Mary, Countess of Bradford and Peter Robertson.

Facing page, Dave Dee, Neil Edmonstone, Justin de Villeneuve (Nigel Stokes), Noel d'Abo, Anthea Norman-Taylor, Tony Bramwell, Stuart Hornall, Jeffery Bridge, Nancy Jarratt and Ray Coleman.

Towards independence

Meanwhile, back at Roehampton, all was not well, much to Sybil's disappointment. She was concerned that the programme should remain a 'Nordoff-Robbins' training, with Roehampton purely providing a certification for the purposes of official recognition, as well as the space for training and therapy. The authorities at Roehampton saw things evolving differently; since the programme was now reliant on the facilities provided by Southlands, should it not be formally adopted by Roehampton Institute? But Sybil's big worry was that, out of the hands of qualified Nordoff-Robbins music therapists, the programme would be vulnerable to institutional development that might dilute or alter the core teaching of Paul and Clive. The tensions arose fairly soon after Nordoff-Robbins' arrival at Southlands, and it quickly became clear that there were irreconcilable differences.

Around the same time it also became apparent that the Nordoff-Robbins fund-raisers, still known as the Junior Fund-Raising Committee (of the Music Therapy Charity) had vastly outgrown their parent organisation, with total profits from music industry events topping £100,000 by the end of their third year. In 1980 an amicable separation from the Music Therapy Charity was made formally, and Nordoff-Robbins became incorporated as a Registered Charity (No. 280960) in its own right in August that year (a lengthy process masterminded by Sam Alder).

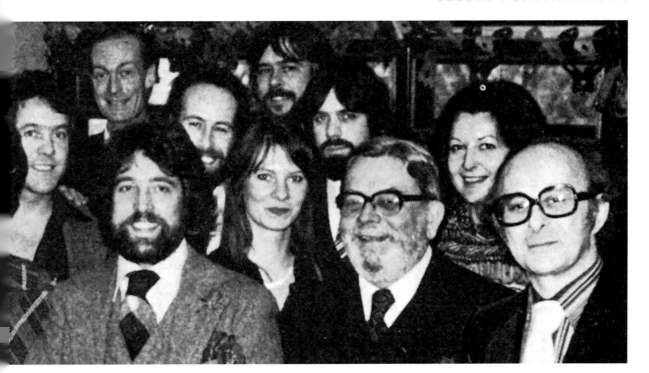

Ian

Ian was in his 40s when a severe asthma attack caused him to suffer oxygen starvation, leading to severe brain damage. He was admitted to a specialist rehabilitation unit, blind and totally paralysed, except for his head, which he could move only a little. He often seemed to be trying to speak, but could not control his mouth enough to make clear sounds. Because Ian had no means of communicating, staff at the unit did not know how much his injury had affected his thinking and understanding.

A Nordoff-Robbins outreach project ran at the rehabilitation unit and Ian was taken to see the music therapist. The therapist began the first session by singing a simple melody. Immediately Ian began vocalising, extending and developing the melody as he laughed and grinned. He began to exchange musical phrases with the therapist. Despite his condition, this was something in which he could participate on an equal basis. Music gave Ian immediate access to a means of communicating and sharing experience. Within a few seconds it had been clearly established that he was in many ways perfectly capable and aware. This gave him the motivation to engage in other therapies, and alerted other staff on the unit to his potential.

The effects of Ian's brain injury meant that he had great difficulty initiating social contact and this increased his isolation. However, after a few weeks of music therapy sessions, Ian started to sing when people entered his bay on the ward as a way of engaging them in interaction. This greatly increased his control of situations and his capacity to form relationships.

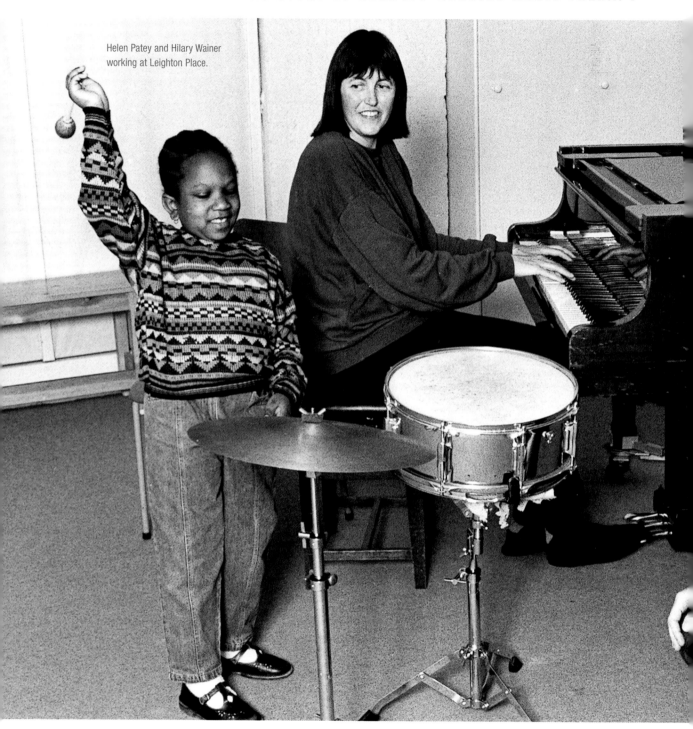

Helen Patey and Hilary Wainer
working at Leighton Place.

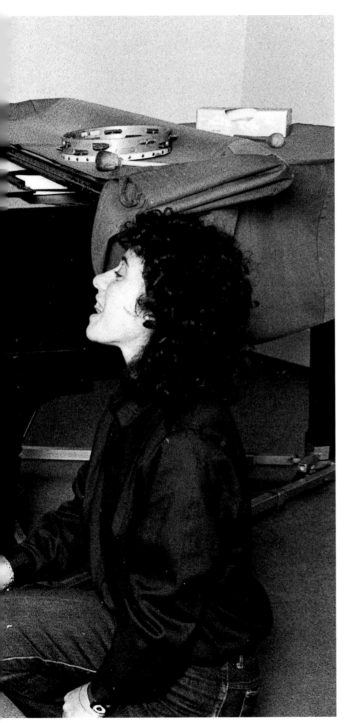

The Centre at Leighton Place, NW5

The association with Roehampton only lasted for three academic years. From an early stage the search was on for a new home, where an independent centre could be established. It was in the late spring of 1981 that a disused wartime small arms factory in Kentish Town, north London was found by a colleague of Sam Alder, who was developing property interests in London. It was a solid, brick building, about 100 years old, in need of major renovation. Jean Elsler was among those searching for suitable premises:

> We [Sybil and I] unlocked and opened the narrow door and were almost overwhelmed by the smell of diesel oil! But it was a very large, empty space leading directly off the street, and we both looked at each other and exclaimed, 'Wonderful!' and that was it. There were just three concrete-floored storeys linked by a twisted,

Jacqueline Robarts working with a physically and mentally disabled woman in her late 20s.

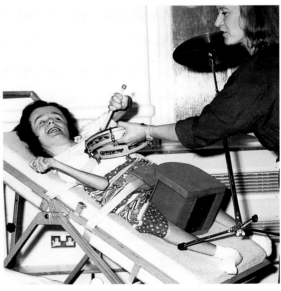

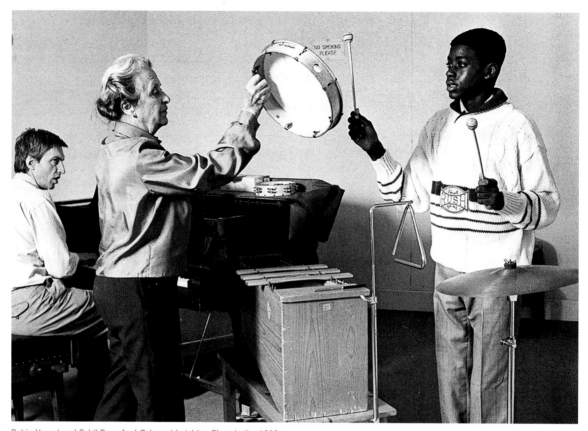

Robin Howat and Sybil Beresford-Peirse at Leighton Place in the 1980s.

narrow staircase, and the top floor was open to the rafters. We just said, 'Gosh, this is wonderful.' Compared to any of the little pokey things we'd seen before it was marvellous.

The building was bought in June 1981 for £50,000, from an endowment fund, with a further £50,000 earmarked for renovation and conversion. Three months later the first Administrator, Rosemary Ward (later Evans), moved in – with just a desk, telephone and mobile gas heater. The builders were hard at work, preparing the new Centre for occupancy in January 1982. Meanwhile, Sybil and her team vacated

Roehampton in the summer of 1981* and had to endure one 'homeless' term, when the students undertook clinical observation at Goldie Leigh and other sites and went to City University in Islington for lectures and teaching.

The move to Leighton Place in January 1982 was a defining moment as the charity realised its dreams of being independent with its own premises. There were two therapy rooms and space for library, administrative and teaching facilities – a lavish provision compared to what they had begun with at Goldie Leigh eight years earlier. The building was officially opened on 3 June 1982 by HRH The Duchess of Gloucester who had taken a keen interest in the work for some years.

* A swift exit became necessary since the music department at Roehampton decided to continue running its own training programme in music therapy. This, like the two existing UK trainings, developed its own unique identity and

approach and was led initially by Elaine Streeter, a student on the first Nordoff-Robbins programme in 1974.

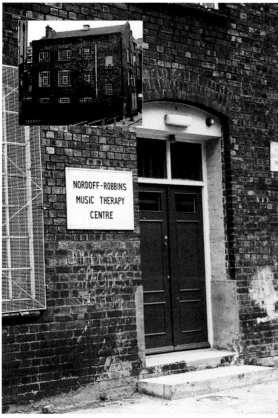

Leighton Place.

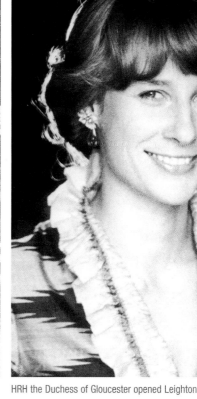

HRH the Duchess of Gloucester opened Leighton Place in 1982.

By now there were a good number of Nordoff-Robbins-trained music therapists (about 50 by 1981) and the expansion of space enabled a few of them to gain employment at the Centre, as therapists or tutors. Jane Gibson, Robin Howat and Rachel Verney all began teaching on the programme around this time. Among the group of students who trained on the first full programme at the new Centre (1982/83) was Pauline Etkin, who was later to follow Sybil as Director. Clive and Carol's input had by now evolved into an annual visit, during which they spent time with the students, presenting case material, teaching group work and watching the students' own clinical work. Sybil, who had found it hard initially to accept Carol as Clive's new partner, became deeply appreciative of her, recognising the strength of her teamwork with Clive. In 1983 Carol was awarded an honorary Nordoff-Robbins diploma from London in appreciation of her contribution to the students' training.

As the Centre became established, relationships with some of the original schools were maintained and more were forged in the new catchment area. The Centre acquired a minibus to bring in schoolchildren from surrounding areas. Margaret Midson joined the staff in May 1986 as Administrator, a post she would hold until her retirement in 2004, providing invaluable support to Sybil and later to

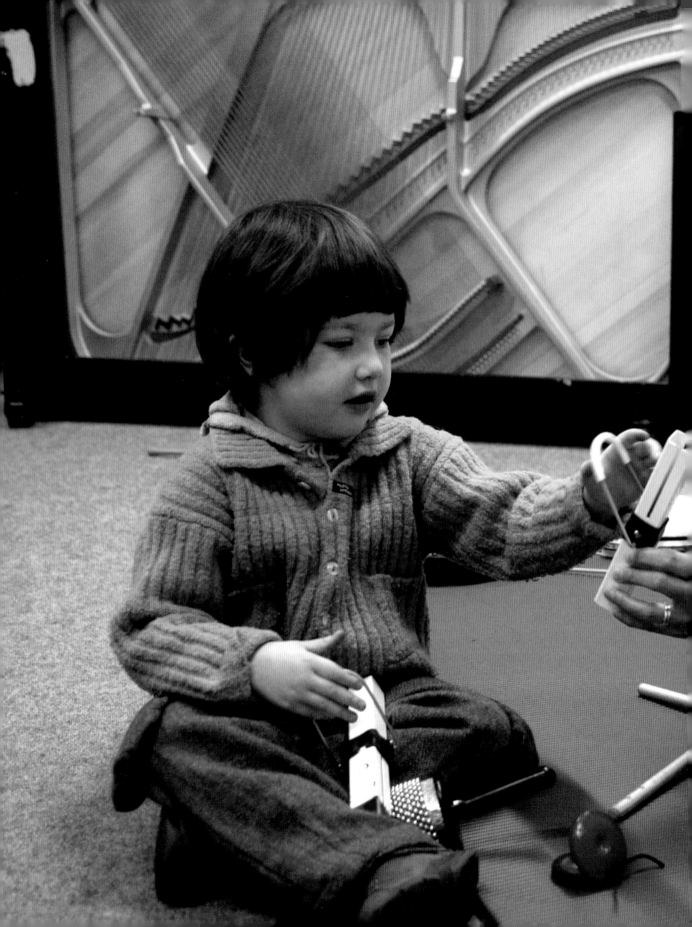

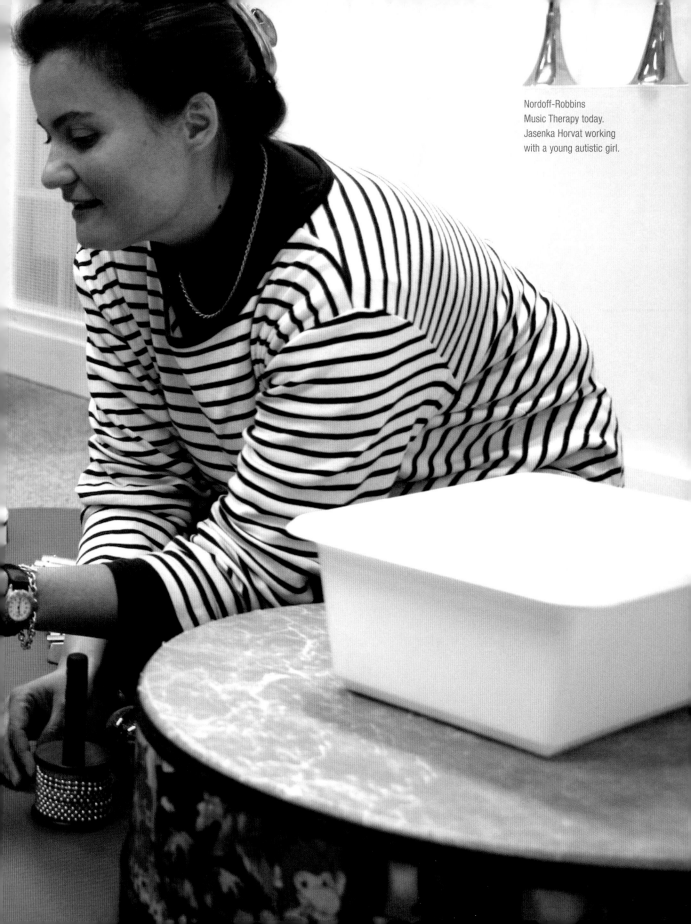

Nordoff-Robbins
Music Therapy today.
Jasenka Horvat working
with a young autistic girl.

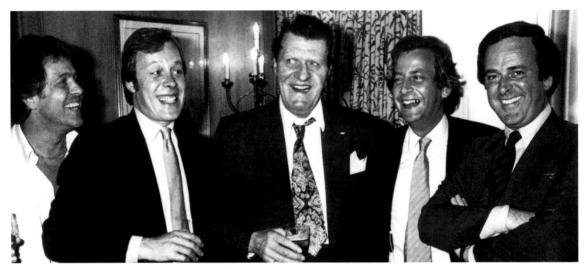

At the 1981 Silver Clef Lunch, left to right, Dave Dee, Willie Robertson, Tommy Cooper, Andrew Miller and Terry Wogan.

Pauline as she ensured the day-to-day smooth operation of the Centre. Meanwhile, the Silver Clef Lunch and other fund-raising activities continued, bringing in the resources that made it all possible. Sybil was enormously grateful for the rock industry funds that were raised. She spoke powerfully and persuasively at the Lunches and was in constant contact with her fund-raisers; yet it would be true to say that the rock-music industry was a disorientating new world for Sybil,

as Nancy Jarratt remembered: 'It seemed a most unlikely alliance between the music industry and one formidable, indomitable lady in her 60s, and it would be true to say that Sybil was bewitched and bewildered by her fund-raisers, their exuberance, their informality, the noisy chaos of our meetings awash with champagne.' And yet there was an extraordinary bond, and across the gaping divisions of age and culture, Sybil had the warm and unending respect of her fund-raisers.

Margaret Midson, Centre Administrator for 18 years.

Steve Stanton, Dean of Validation at City University, second right, with music therapists, left to right: Yid-Ee Goh, Claire Threlfall, Evangeline Kai-Wen Cheng and Wyomia Goveya graduating in 2003.

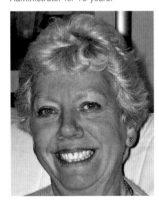

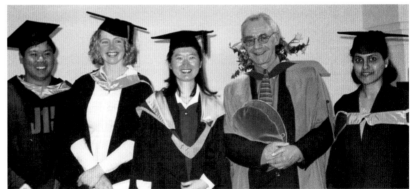

Perhaps it was because she belonged to an utterly different world from the one they inhabited that they were so devoted to enabling her to carry out her mission.

City University

The immediate disadvantage of leaving Roehampton was that the training programme was temporarily thrown back into the vulnerable state of being uncertified by an academic institution. Sybil knew Malcolm Troup at City University (through the Music Therapy Charity, of which he was a Governor), and she was already in dialogue with him at Roehampton about the possibility of City University validating the Nordoff-Robbins training. The resulting collaboration was City University's first venture of this nature and has been a fruitful relationship for both parties, serving as a prototype for many more validation relationships between City University and other institutions in later years, including various performing arts and psychotherapeutic applications.

Steve Stanton, a music lecturer (later Dean of Validation) became the key architect of the collaboration, negotiating at length with Sybil and the University to provide an endorsement with which both institutions would be happy. This was no mean task, since the University initially wanted five three-hour written papers, while Sybil wanted none (music therapy training is first and foremost a practical course). To this day, Steve chairs the Nordoff-Robbins Course Board and is a wise, supportive guide for the education and training programmes within the charity.

The process of gaining validation proved extremely lengthy, requiring the endorsement of the Board of Studies in Music and Senate (City University's governing body), as well as external assessors. Sybil became understandably frustrated with the process because she wanted her students to be armed with a proper qualification, and the

City University

The City University at Northampton Square, EC1, was only a short distance from the Nordoff-Robbins Music Therapy Centre at Leighton Place. More importantly, its music department had an ethos that fitted perfectly with music therapy. Historically, the university had been founded to offer professional training in science and technology, closely associated with industry and commerce. In this environment a unique BSc Music degree course had been established in the mid-1970s that attempted to bridge the gap between music as science and music as art, masterminded by Wilfrid Mellers of York University and Malcolm Troup of the Guildhall School of Music and Drama who ultimately became Professor of Music at City University.

Unlike a standard university music degree, teaching 'pure' music, the City course attempted to link music to other disciplines, offering modules on psychological, biological, physiological and sociological aspects of music-making, together with music technology and ethnomusicology, while also linking up with the Guildhall for conservatoire performance tuition.

As Professor of Music, Malcolm Troup established a Research Fellowship in Music Therapy at City University in 1981, supported by the Music Therapy Charity (and for many years by Nordoff-Robbins), and when Sybil looked for institutional certification of the Nordoff-Robbins course, City University was the obvious place to turn.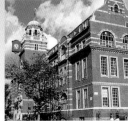

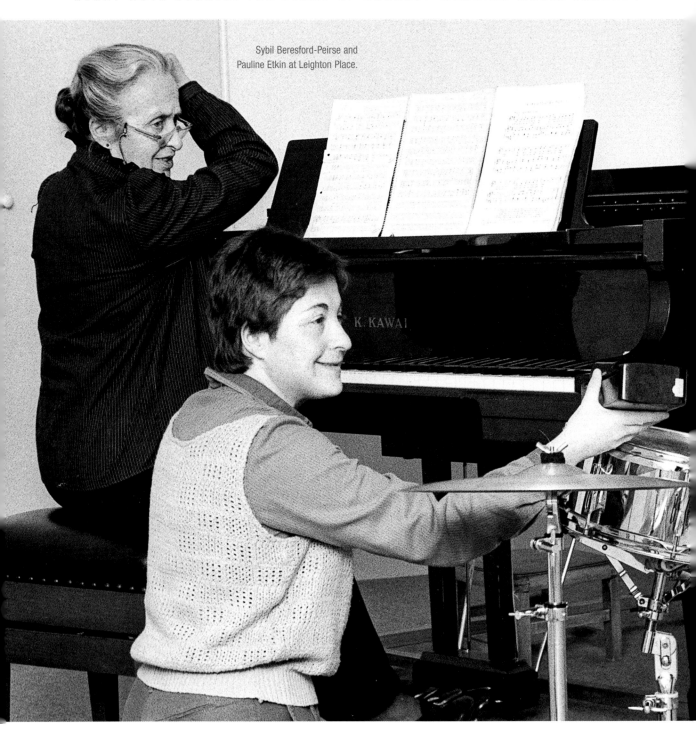

Sybil Beresford-Peirse and
Pauline Etkin at Leighton Place.

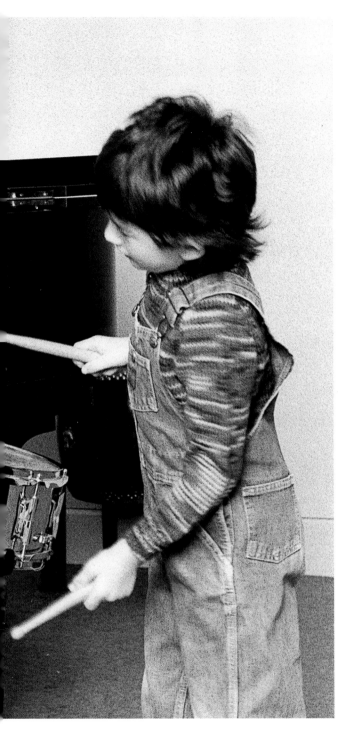

validation was also necessary for students to obtain grants. Her protestations notwithstanding, the process ran a proper course, and on 19 October 1983 the training programme was finally validated by City University Senate. The validation agreement was signed in March 1984, with an initial validation period of three years. It was therefore in the summer of 1984 that the first graduates were awarded the City University Diploma, although the validation was back-dated to allow the students who had finished in 1982 and 1983 to receive the City University qualification as well. It was a tremendously important milestone for Nordoff-Robbins Music Therapy. With independent premises for therapy and training, and a university-validated programme, Nordoff-Robbins had truly come of age.

Through the years the relationship with City has remained constant. Today it is difficult for the university to validate a course with fewer than 100 students, since there must be a minimum critical mass to make it financially viable. With an average intake of six students each year, Nordoff-Robbins has a special relationship with City University.

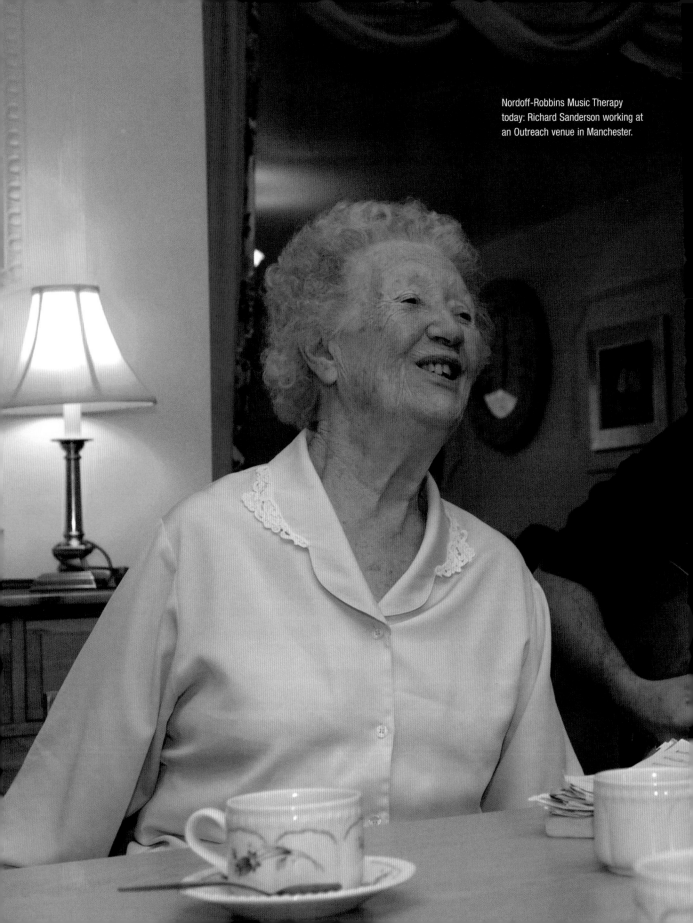

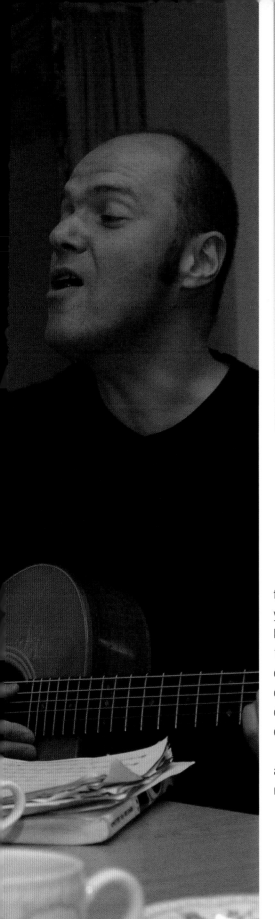

4 Coming of Age

By the early 1980s Nordoff-Robbins had gained status as an independent registered charity; it had its own Centre at Leighton Place, a successful fund-raising organisation and a university-validated training programme. All this was a remarkable achievement in less than ten years since the birth of the charity. Meanwhile, the number of Nordoff-Robbins graduates increased steadily each year, rising from 43 in 1980 to 121 in 1990. The 1980s saw the beginning of rapid development of the work outside the Centre in various parts of the country, including a wide expansion of clinical fields. Some of the work was funded by the Nordoff-Robbins charity, while in other places it was established independently by graduates of the training programme.

Among the early music therapists who adopted the Nordoff-Robbins approach, Julienne Cartwright (née Brown) (1928–98), a South African national, deserves particular mention as the first person to apply it in working

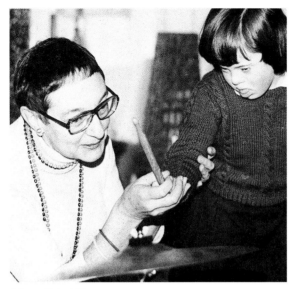

Julienne Cartwright.

she read Nordoff and Robbins' first book. Within moments of meeting Sybil in 1972 she was appointed Secretary of the Nordoff-Robbins Project Committee, when Sybil discovered she could type. Jean began working with Sybil at Goldie Leigh Hospital and trained on the first programme in 1974. When the programme moved to Roehampton in 1978 Jean maintained the service at Goldie Leigh as Head of Department, and many newly-qualified therapists went to work with her to gain experience. Here, and at Queen Mary's Hospital for Children in Surrey where she established a Music Therapy Department in 1984, Jean led many creative developments in the Nordoff-Robbins work. An outstanding inspiration to generations of music therapy students, since her retirement from Queen Mary's in 1991 Jean has continued to practice and teach at the Nordoff-Robbins Centre, maintaining extraordinary youthful vigour.

Nordoff-Robbins Music Therapy continued to thrive in a number of special schools in London, most notably Sybil Elgar School, Harborough School and Richard Cloudesley School. It also took root in other parts of the country, such as

with adults. A fellow student of Sybil on the first Guildhall programme, Julienne was a person of great vision and determination, who began the work at Goldie Leigh Hospital before her marriage in 1973 took her to East Lothian in Scotland. At Haddington, encouraged by Paul Nordoff, she gained employment at the adult psychiatric facility, Herdmanflat Hospital, and at East Fortune Hospital, where she worked with adults with learning disabilities and older people with dementia. Later on Julienne was joined by other therapists in the establishment of Nordoff-Robbins Scotland in the 1980s, but for eight years she ploughed on alone. Through her regular visits to London to speak to the Nordoff-Robbins trainees, and later as the external examiner, Julienne influenced a whole generation of therapists, who were to apply Nordoff-Robbins principles in new clinical areas.

Equal mention must be made of Jean Eisler, whose association with Nordoff-Robbins spans the duration of the charity's existence and who has been a key figure in its development. Like Sybil, Jean encountered music therapy later in life, when

Jean Eisler at the concert given at the Nordoff-Robbins Centre to celebrate her 90th birthday, April 2006.

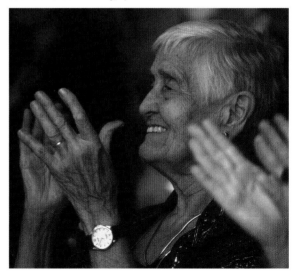

Queen Mary's Hospital and Orchard Hill

In the early 1980s Queen Mary's Hospital for Children in Surrey provided specialist services for children, including those with emotional-behavioural problems, psychiatric disorders and learning disabilities. A large residential facility, Orchard Hill, Carshalton, had just been built for young adults with learning disabilities who had lived all their lives on the long-stay children's wards.

In 1982 an innovative full-time music therapy post was created at Orchard Hill and Jacqueline Robarts began working there, inspired by Julienne Cartwright's work in Scotland. Her work generated great interest across the Queen Mary's site, and in 1984 Jean Eisler began running a small department of three music therapists, part-funded by Nordoff-Robbins. For seven years Jean presided over the team, with the range of referrals constantly extending the therapists' clinical skills and musical creativity. Jacqueline became Head of Department for three years when Jean retired in 1991; during this time she negotiated with the NHS to fund the posts, and responded to the changing service framework by steering the department into two separate music therapy services (adults and children) which continue to thrive today.

Ravenswood Village, Berkshire

Ravenswood Village was founded in 1953 by four Jewish families who each had a child with a learning disability and wanted to improve the level of care for their children. Set in 120 acres of Berkshire countryside, this residential community is home to 175 people. It is an impressive example of the kind of provision that can be created for people with learning disabilities, enabling them to live life to the full and gain maximum independence. Sybil Beresford-Peirse organised visits for her students from the early years of the training programme; the contact was forged through Dr Franz Morgenstern, who was an Honorary Consultant Psychiatrist at Ravenswood and a member of Sybil's first Nordoff-Robbins committee in 1971. At least 17 Nordoff-Robbins therapists have worked at Ravenswood since 1978.

London Lighthouse

London Lighthouse opened in 1988 in west London as Britain's first major residential and support centre for people living with HIV and AIDS. Funded by Nordoff-Robbins Music Therapy, Colin Lee began a music therapy service at London Lighthouse in 1989. As a little-explored clinical area for music therapists, it quickly became apparent that the potency of the work in facilitating expressions of health and life is as relevant to people with a terminal diagnosis as any, if not more so. Colin's work at Lighthouse provided clinical material for his doctoral research at City University and paved the way for a second generation of Nordoff-Robbins-trained therapists, including Nigel Hartley and Nicky O'Neill, to develop music therapy work with people with life-threatening illness and in palliative care.

North Yorkshire and Ravenswood Village in Berkshire, and by the end of the 1980s the work had expanded into a wide range of clinical fields.

Developments at Leighton Place

The Centre in Kentish Town quickly generated interest in the local community and demand for therapy grew rapidly. In 1984 Jean Eisler established a clinic at the Centre on Saturdays; this service employed several therapists and soon became one of the busiest days.

Sybil Beresford-Peirse was now in her early 70s, and though she remained indomitable, City University was concerned that, as Head of Training, her age was in fact in breach of university regulations. It was towards the end of 1985 when the university finally told Sybil she would have to retire. She was bitterly resentful, as she wanted to continue, but the position was untenable. Sybil's role in the establishment of Nordoff-Robbins had been absolutely central and her achievement immense, but it was right that a younger generation should now be allowed to develop the training programme in response to the changing needs of students

North Yorkshire Music Therapy Centre

One enterprising early graduate of the Nordoff-Robbins training programme (1977-78), Mary Abbotson, established a private practice in Kirkbymoorside, North Yorkshire in 1984. As the only music therapy service in the area it quickly attracted county-wide interest, and in order to better meet the needs of the rural community a Mobile Music Therapy Unit was introduced in 1989. This custom built van, designed by her husband and team-mate Raymond, contained a digital piano and full range of musical instruments for use in therapy. The van was fitted with insulation, ventilation, electric lighting, heating, cupboards and even a sink supplied with hot water.

The space provided an excellent venue for individual work and allowed for groups of up to five children. The mobile unit had significant advantages over the traditional spaces in schools and hospitals where music therapists might work. It was flexible and cost-effective, and nobody need be refused music therapy for lack of suitable space or resources. Setting up was quick and the space was free from the distractions of schools and the interruptions to which sessions in such environments are inevitably prone. The van also provided its own effective advertising, proclaiming *The North Yorkshire Music Therapy Centre* in large letters as it roamed around the county.

Generous financial support was received from Tyne Tees Telethon and Children in Need, enabling the service to expand,

encompassing not only children with special needs, but also the elderly and adults with mental health problems. Two later substantial grants from the Headley Trust gave rise to some innovative collaborative research with York University into electronic instruments and tools for the therapists' analysis of sessions.

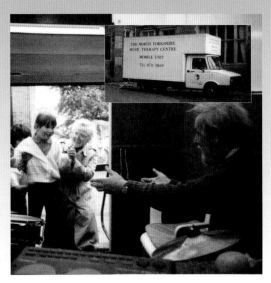

and the profession. Sybil took it very hard and, though no longer Head of Training, she remained Director of the Centre for a further five years.

During these five years Sybil presided over two Heads of Training, both of whom had a challenging time with Sybil supervising them. Alyson Carter was appointed in 1986 and was succeeded two years later by Robin Howat. Their job was made somewhat easier by the acquisition of several venues in the vicinity of the Centre where teaching could take place, but it remained a difficult situation, as Robin remembered:

It was difficult because she [Sybil] didn't want to let go. Having the premises at Carker's Lane helped, just by being physically absent [from Leighton Place], but she would be very much wanting to take back the reins. It was always a jostle . . . She still came in on some teaching. She tried very hard to be good about it, I think. She really had good intentions but they would be overridden by her desire to be in there.

Robin's leadership of the training programme saw a loosening of the close adherence to the original 1974 recordings of Paul Nordoff, which had continued to be used by Sybil as a central focus of the programme structure. Students were still encouraged to listen to the tapes, but a greater spirit of enquiry was opened up so that the teaching sessions could be better adapted to the learning needs of individual students. Robin held this post until his departure for Australia in 1993.

Lissenden Gardens: a new Centre

As the training programme developed, so clinical work at the Centre simultaneously continued to flourish and grow. By 1987 the hunt was on again for new premises that would enable further expansion, as Leighton Place had limited space and the demand for therapy was growing. Once again, it was Sam Alder who eventually found the perfect site, less than a mile away, in Lissenden Gardens, beside Hampstead Heath.

The building was a disused power station: a massive, brick, shed-like structure built in the 1890s for generating electricity from coal and now little more than a storehouse full of disused heavy machinery. The only real hazard was a huge electrical transformer inside, which would need to be rehoused. The owner of the property lived in the top floor of the Regency period house, 175 Highgate Road, which stood right in front of the old power station, and there were three further flats in this building. It was clear that the two buildings together would make a fantastic suite, with the house providing valuable extra space for living quarters and teaching. Though the house was not for sale at the outset, fortunately the owner was later persuaded to part with it.

The power station was purchased for £700,000 in July 1988 on a large bank loan. The architects, Sampson Associates, were employed to design the conversion, and the London Electricity Board agreed to the repositioning of the electrical transformer in a shed to be erected at the side of the building. The whole venture was an ambitious conception, and Pauline Etkin and Robin Howat worked closely with Sybil (whose health was failing) and the architects, particularly Douglas Binnie, in developing a design. Today it remains the largest purpose-designed centre for music therapy in the world: a spacious three-floor structure, with three sound-proofed therapy rooms, each with an observation booth, a large conference hall; and extensive teaching facilities.

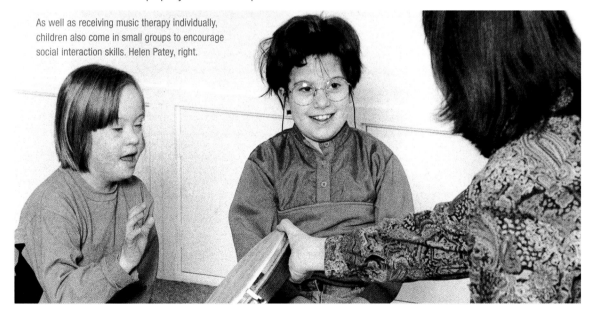

As well as receiving music therapy individually, children also come in small groups to encourage social interaction skills. Helen Patey, right.

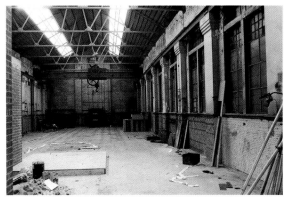

The power station at Lissenden Gardens before its transformation into the new Nordoff-Robbins Music Therapy Centre, *right*.

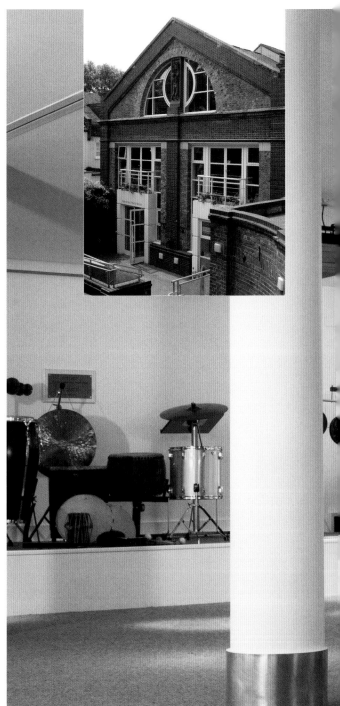

Knebworth

The renovation and conversion of Lissenden Gardens was to cost in the region of £3 million. This was serious money by any standards, and the fund-raising team took up the challenge. Their brilliant idea was to hold a massive open-air concert, bringing together all the Silver Clef Award winners from the past 14 years. For many, the concert at Knebworth Park in Hertfordshire on 30 June 1990 was the most exciting event in the history of Nordoff-Robbins fund-raising – certainly the most ambitious. The day-long concert was a huge feat of organisation and took two years to plan, from the summer of 1988 when Andrew Miller first began speaking to the band managers. Paul McCartney, who was presented with the Silver Clef Award in 1988, was the first act to confirm, and from then on the accept-ances rolled in – Status Quo, Genesis, Phil Collins, Eric Clapton, Tears For Fears, Dire Straits, Pink Floyd, Elton John, Robert Plant and Jimmy Page, and Cliff Richard and The Shadows.

The success of Knebworth exceeded everybody's wildest dreams. The concert sold out and became one of most celebrated events in rock history. The musicians played to a live audience of 120,000 music fans, and it was broadcast simultaneously around the world on MTV, which paid its

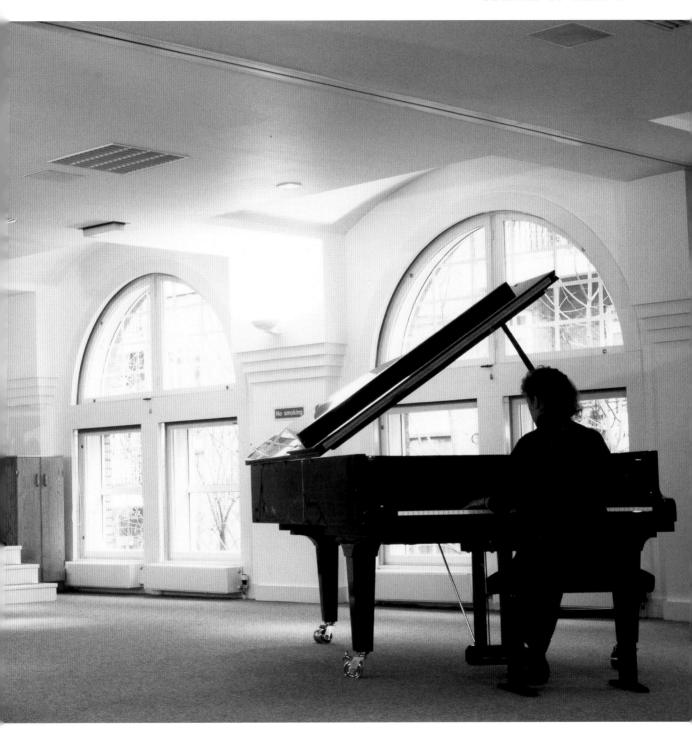

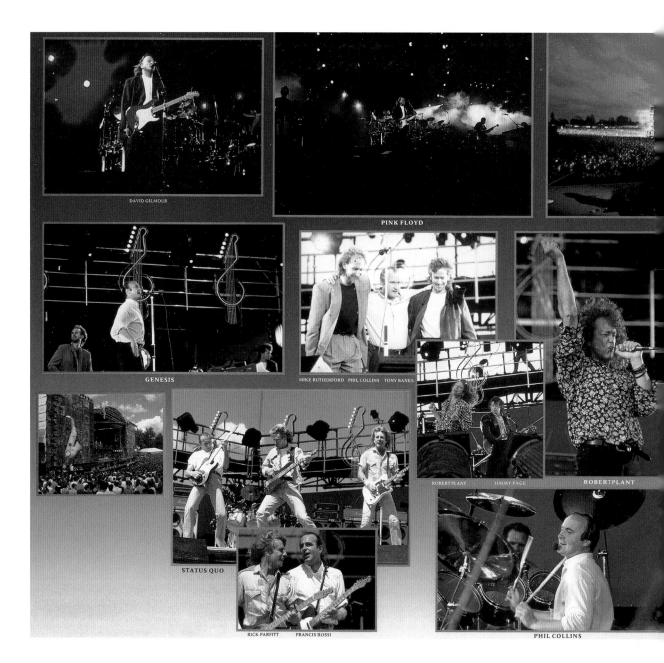

DAVID GILMOUR

PINK FLOYD

GENESIS

MIKE RUTHERFORD   PHIL COLLINS   TONY BANKS

ROBERT PLANT   JIMMY PAGE

ROBERT PLANT

STATUS QUO

RICK PARFITT   FRANCIS ROSSI

PHIL COLLINS

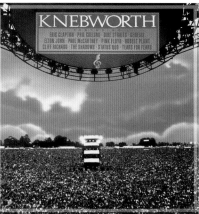

Left and above, front cover and inside of the LP record of the Knebworth Concert, June 1990, in aid of Nordoff-Robbins and the BRIT Trust.

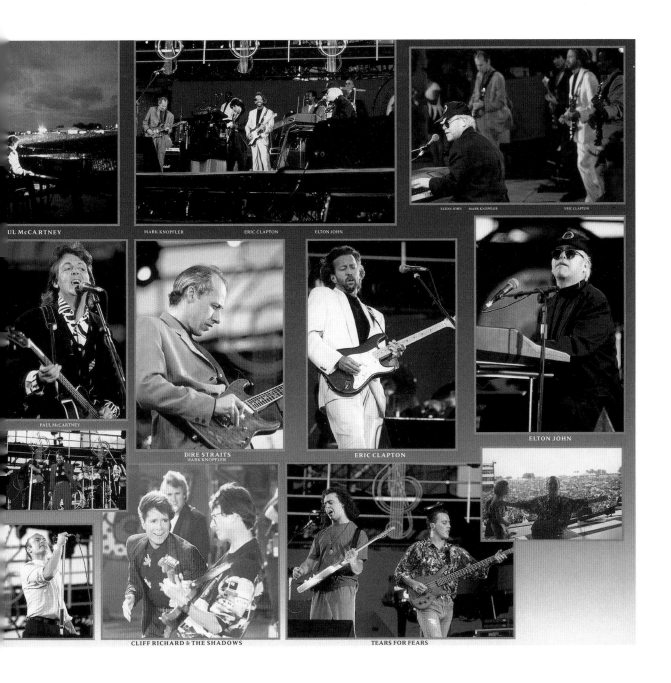

UL McCARTNEY   MARK KNOPFLER   ERIC CLAPTON   ELTON JOHN

ELTON JOHN   MARK KNOPFLER   ERIC CLAPTON

PAUL McCARTNEY

DIRE STRAITS
MARK KNOPFLER

ERIC CLAPTON

ELTON JOHN

CLIFF RICHARD & THE SHADOWS   TEARS FOR FEARS

Knebworth's most enduring legacy was that the best rock musicians in the world considered music therapy a force to be reckoned with, worthy of their time and support.

biggest fee ever to cover the event. The *Daily Mail* ran a four-page spread about the concert, and critics hailed it an historic occasion, dubbing it 'The Dinosaurs of Rock' for showcasing the best of British rock music from the previous two decades. For some acts it was a rare appearance – Pink Floyd gave their only live performance that year, while Cliff Richard and the Shadows came together to perform for the first time in six years. The final heavy downpour of rain under which performers and fans shared the occasion added to the drama and uniqueness of the experience. Even today the Knebworth

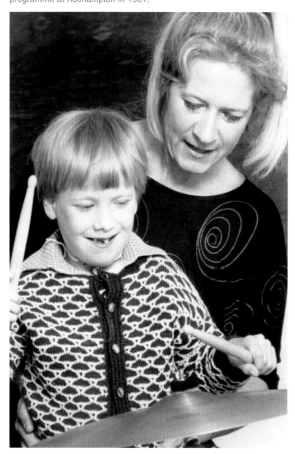

Jacqueline Robarts qualified from the training programme at Roehampton in 1981.

concert is remembered as an almost legendary event, and the successful release of the concert on DVD in 2002 testifies to the enduring memory of the occasion among diehard rock fans.

Profits from Knebworth totalled well over £6 million with the inclusion of royalties arising from the worldwide best-seller album *Knebworth 90* which was recorded at the concert. Nordoff-Robbins got its new Centre and shared the proceeds which enabled the BRIT Trust to establish their School for Performing Arts and Technology in Croydon. But apart from the superb new premises, perhaps Knebworth's most enduring legacy for Nordoff-Robbins was the symbolic significance of reaching the consciousness of a world audience and the entire international music industry. The underlying message was that the best rock musicians in the world considered music therapy a force to be reckoned with, worthy of their time and support. Knebworth demonstrated the British music industry's continuing commitment to Nordoff-Robbins and ensured that this unique alliance would go on into the future.

The opening of the Centre

Sam Alder's property company was appointed to manage the construction project at Lissenden Gardens, and Sam generously donated the time and expertise of his project manager, Margaret Baxter, to oversee the work. Problems arose when the building contractors went into liquidation but the new Centre was ready by the summer of 1991. With great celebration, the building was formally opened on 25 September by the Duchess of York, who had taken an interest in the work and had visited the old Centre at Leighton Place in March 1989.

Sybil took this historic moment as her time to finally retire. The accolades that she received for her services to music therapy, including an OBE in 1985, were richly deserved. Had she been a less exacting taskmaster, it is probable that the

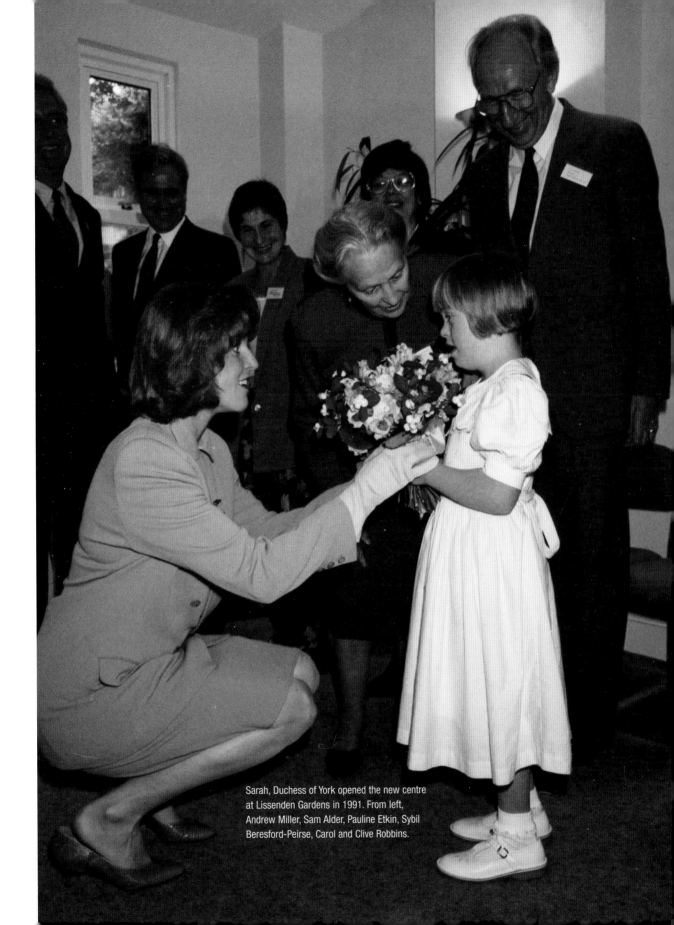

Sarah, Duchess of York opened the new centre at Lissenden Gardens in 1991. From left, Andrew Miller, Sam Alder, Pauline Etkin, Sybil Beresford-Peirse, Carol and Clive Robbins.

Grace

Grace lived with an ongoing schizophrenic illness; like many people suffering with a chronic mental health illness, she alternated periods of hospitalisation with her life outside. On average, Grace was admitted to hospital (usually against her will) several times a year, and whenever she was there she had sessions with the resident music therapist. She sang songs about her life, gospel songs about her love of her family and friends, and God.

Grace said that music was the one thing in hospital that made her feel human. A place of enjoyment and warmth, and a haven from intrusive thoughts, music somehow connected the strands of her life when the force of her illness seemed to be unravelling it. It was a vital part of her inpatient treatment programme.

power station was purchased and converted to serve several functions: it housed a boardroom for the fund-raising committee, as well as the Director's apartment, and later became the main teaching space for the training programme. The house was named after Lady Bradford, Sybil's vivacious and close friend, who had been responsible for first introducing the Music Therapy Charity to Andrew Miller, who established the all important fund-raising link with the rock industry. Mary Bradford had continued to work tirelessly for Nordoff-Robbins in her capacity as Honorary Chairman of the Junior Fund-Raising Committee. Her death in 1986 was a personal loss for many people involved with the Nordoff-Robbins charity, and the inauguration of Mary Bradford House became a fitting tribute.

Life at the new Centre

As the largest purpose-built music therapy centre in the world, the opening of Lissenden Gardens in 1991 marked a new era, not only for Nordoff-Robbins Music Therapy, but for the profession in Britain as a whole. Pauline Etkin, who had supported Sybil through the years leading up to her retirement, now became Director. She was keen to open the doors of the new spacious facilities to all music therapists and other related professionals, so that as many people as

Nordoff-Robbins Music Therapy charity would not exist today; in her own words, she had to be 'as tough as an old boot' to achieve all that she did.*

The Regency period house that stood in front of the old

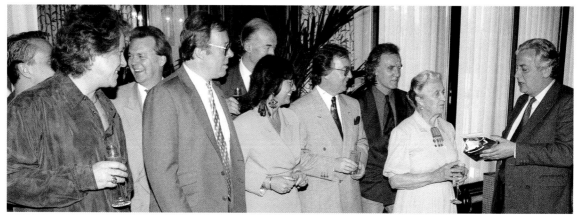

Andrew Miller making a presentation to Sybil Beresford-Peirse at her retirement party at the Inter-Continental Hotel, 1991. Left to right, Curt Smith of Tears for Fears (partly hidden), Dave Dee, Steve Smith, Willie Robertson, Neil Edmonstone, Audrey Hoare, Neil Warnock and Bob Young.

* When Sybil died 11 years later, days short of her 90th birthday in 2002, the main Centre building was renamed Beresford-Peirse House in recognition of her achievement in establishing a permanent legacy in England of Paul Nordoff and Clive Robbins' pioneering work.

Pauline Etkin

Pauline Etkin, who trained on the 1982/83 programme, came to music therapy, like Sybil Beresford-Peirse, with a background in teacher training. In the years immediately after qualifying she worked as a music therapist in London and in her native South Africa, before settling permanently in London in 1986 when she was offered a teaching and therapy post at the Nordoff-Robbins Centre. Two years later she became Assistant Director of the Centre, at the same time as Robin Howat became Head of Training, and she succeeded Sybil as Director in 1991. On Robin's departure in 1993, the posts of Director and Head of Training were recombined and Pauline held this position for ten years before becoming Managing Director of Nordoff-Robbins Music Therapy in 2002 as part of the management restructure.

Pauline Etkin brought a different style of leadership to Nordoff-Robbins in her role as Director: one that was more collaborative and offered her staff a greater degree of autonomy and creative contribution than they had known previously. Over 16 years she has been an energetic, sensitive and effective leader, offering wise direction through the steady growth of the charity's many activities.

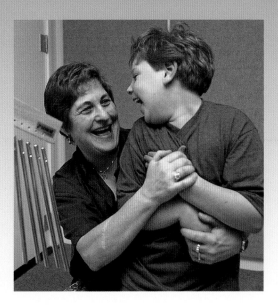

possible could benefit from its resources. The Centre became a locus for professional activity: the two nationwide music therapy associations, the Association of Professional Music Therapists (APMT) and the British Society for Music Therapy (BSMT), were invited to make regular use of the Centre for conferences and meetings, and students from other training programmes visited to use library facilities and observe sessions in progress. A spirit of open dialogue and cross-fertilisation was fostered. A number of Centre staff members have undertaken committee roles within the APMT and BSMT over the years, which has also contributed to the developing cooperation between the Centre and the wider music therapy profession. Among them, Helen Patey served as BSMT Chairperson (1994–98); Nigel Hartley as BSMT Chairperson (1998–2002) and as APMT Chairperson (2002–04); and Judith Nockolds as APMT Chairperson (2004–2007).

The increased space for clinical work quickly led to increased demand, and soon around 150 children and adults were being seen for music therapy at the Centre every week. The untimely death of David Morris in 1989 left the Board of Governors without a Chairman; Sybil became Acting Chairman for two years before the position was taken up in 1991 by Professor Joan Bicknell, Professor of the Psychiatry of Mental Handicap at St George's Hospital Medical School, London. With her breadth of professional experience, Joan Bicknell was ideally suited to the role. She presided for six years, expecting high standards of practice within the Centre and making a significant contribution to its development by her sensitive guidance through the transition. She was succeeded in 1997 by Sam Alder, whose invaluable support for the charity throughout its existence has been mentioned already.

Development of training and research

In 1993 Pauline Etkin became Head of Training in addition to being Director of the Centre. She gathered around her a strong team of therapists to manage the programme. Julie Allis, as Course Tutor, taught the core clinical studies and supervised group work until she moved to the USA in spring 1996; Sandra Brown became Clinical Coordinator, introducing a new system of individual supervision and heading the team of clinical supervisors who oversaw the students' own clinical work; Jane Gibson continued to develop the musical resources and clinical improvisation teaching until 2005; Helen Patey, in addition to

her clinical management as Assistant Director of the Centre (later Deputy Managing Director), expanded the teaching of group work to students; Julia Usher took over from Jenny Purvis the teaching of group improvisation; Sarah Verney Caird and Nigel Hartley pioneered personal individual music therapy for the students on the training programme. Many other music therapists and external lecturers also enriched the training programme with clinical and background studies.

In the mid-1990s the Nordoff-Robbins training programme developed from a one-year diploma into a two-year Master of Music Therapy degree (MMT). This was the fulfilment of a dream that had been taking shape in Pauline Etkin and Steve Stanton's minds for several years, the purpose of the expansion being two-fold: to equip students with research skills to keep pace with the evolving international profession, and secondly to introduce specific training in work with adult clients (a number of

From top left, Helen Patey, Deputy Managing Director and Head of Clinical Services. Heads of departments: Dr Julie Sutton, Training (until 2007); Dr Gary Ansdell and Mercédès Pavlicevic (Co-Heads) Research; Rachel Verney, National Outreach; Donald Wetherick, Publicity. Sandra Brown, Year One Clinical Coordinator; Judith Nockolds, Year Two Clinical Coordinator; Jacqueline Robarts, Musical Resources Tutor; Oksana Zharinova-Sanderson, Regional Head, Nordoff-Robbins Music Therapy North West; Nicky O'Neill, Therapist in charge of Saturdays; Simon Procter, Programme Director from 2007.

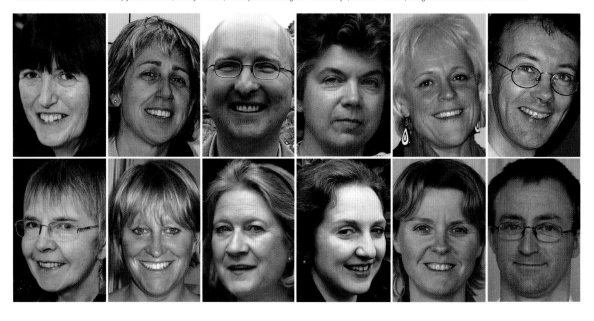

graduates were now working in this sphere, but the diploma programme still focused exclusively on work with children with special needs).

Gary Ansdell, a graduate of the 1987/88 course, was invited by Pauline to become Year Two Coordinator. Gary brought both research skills, as he had gone on to obtain a Master's from the University of Witten-Herdecke, Germany, in 1991, and wide clinical experience with adult clients*. Rachel Verney formed the other half of the team, as Year Two Placement and Supervision Coordinator, and together they formulated the second year curriculum and worked towards a starting date of September 1996 (for the 1995/97 cohort of students). Like Gary, Rachel had also been involved with the German Nordoff-Robbins training programme at Witten-Herdecke, having been part of its early establishment in the late 1970s, and she had many years' experience of working with adults. Mercédès Pavlicevic, who had completed a PhD at Edinburgh University in 1991, after her Nordoff-Robbins training (1980/81), was also drafted in as an advisor, to help devise the curriculum for the research component and the infrastructure for guaranteeing the Master's level standard. Steve Stanton from City University provided the requisite institutional advice, critiquing the curriculum ideas and frameworks for assessment, and ensuring that the necessary safeguards were in place; while Pauline Etkin, as Head of Training, oversaw the balance and overall development of the programme. Relationships were forged with a number of institutions in London for students' clinical placements.

Thus Nordoff-Robbins began offering the first full-time, two-year music therapy training programme in the country. It was a major success, providing a new level of comprehensive preparation for the profession; enabling new graduates to work reflectively, with confidence and innovation, and to contribute authoritatively to the growing body of literature and research in the field.

The establishment of the new Master's degree in 1996 also

* Gary Ansdell made his first major contribution to music therapy literature with *Music for Life* (1995) which was the first book exploring the application of the Nordoff-Robbins Music Therapy approach to adult clients.

Stella

Aged 14, Stella had been battling anorexia nervosa for two years, with episodes of suicidal depression that revealed the turmoil of anxiety that lay beneath her alternately obstreperous and withdrawn behaviour. Stella seemed to be stemming the flow of life in her self-imprisoned world.

During her in-patient admission Stella was referred for music therapy and came with initial reluctance. In an early session, sitting beside the therapist at the treble end of the piano, she listlessly played an endless circling motif that went nowhere, in which the music therapist joined her, providing support. A breakthrough came when, in response to Stella's chromatic harmonies, the therapist started to play 'Over the Rainbow', a song full of hope. Stella's patterns immediately began to take on a different shape, leading to a playful and animated exchange of three-note motifs.

Such moments of sharing and interaction slowly began to diminish Stella's isolation and rigidity of self-expression. Four sessions later, at the therapist's suggestion, she started to sing tentatively and very quietly, reflecting on how she felt about herself, as the therapist improvised music. In subsequent sessions she began to use different songs as metaphors for her states of mind, and explored new places to play: the bass of the piano, and then other instruments around the room – the conga drums, Swanee whistle and kazoo. Now Stella was filling the space with a new vitality and sense of direction, valuing the changes in herself and her music.

Stella experienced herself anew through the immediacy of music and through dynamic, expressive interplay with her therapist, both of which opened new pathways of being, doing, playing and relating. After nine months Stella recovered sufficiently to return home and resume her schooling, continuing music therapy in a group as part of her outpatient support programme.

coincided with the rapid growth of an international music therapy research community, and it was a natural step for the Centre to develop a research profile as well, in response to the growing demand for evidence-based practice. Research had been a key element of the charity's tripartite mandate (therapy, training and research) since the 1980s, and when Gary Ansdell completed his PhD at City University in 1999, this opened new doors in terms of what the Centre could offer. Simon Procter was employed in late 2000 to work as Research Assistant, and a Research Department was set up in 2002, with Gary Ansdell as Head of Research, later to be joined by Mercédès Pavlicevic as Co-Head in 2006. Among many recent developments, the launch in January 2006 of an MPhil/PhD Research Degree programme, in partnership with City University, has contributed significantly to the international profile of the charity.

Structure of the charity today

Andrew Miller retired from his position as Director of Fund-Raising in 2000, after 24 years of outstanding work for the charity. In 1994, he and Willie Robertson were presented with the esteemed Music Industry Trusts Award in recognition of the achievement of their conception and growth of the Nordoff-Robbins Charity. Andrew was succeeded by Audrey Hoare as Director of Fund-Raising. Audrey had worked for the charity since 1989 as Appeals Organiser: she has initiated many new projects and now leads a team of four at the fund-raising office. On Andrew's retirement Derek Green and Jeremy Marsh became Co-Chairmen of the Fund-Raising Committee; each brought a wealth of experience in the music industry, Derek Green as former Managing Director of A&M Records, ex-Director of the British Phonographic Industry and head of China Records, and Jeremy Marsh as Managing Director of Telstar Records. In 2006 there were 43 people working for the Fund-

Raising Committee, of whom only four were salaried employees. Among the original members, Willie Robertson, Sam Alder, Nancy Jarratt and Dave Dee have continued to work tirelessly for the charity to the present day. In 2004 Derek Green and Jeremy Marsh were succeeded by Brian McLaughlin, Chief Operating Officer of HMV Group plc (2001–05). Nordoff-Robbins Music Therapy has been HMV's nominated charity for more than 20 years. Brian McLaughlin's contribution to the music industry has been recognised with many honours, including the Music Week Strat Award in 1996 (previously awarded to Sybil Beresford-Peirse in 1989), the Music Industry Trusts Award in 2001 and the Silver Clef Chairman's Award in 2002. In 2007 Derek Green was appointed Chairman of the Board of Governors in succession to Sam Alder who retired after 32 years of dedicated work for Nordoff-Robbins.

The management structure of the charity received a complete overhaul in 2002, with Pauline Etkin becoming Managing Director. There were several motives for this: first, the developing national profile of the charity required a leadership structure that was less London-based; and second, there was a desire to bring all the activities of the charity under one umbrella, with increased interlinking between therapists and fund-raisers. In addition, a more formalised structure of accountability was needed for an organisation that had by now vastly outgrown its informal, *ad hoc* beginnings. The new structure comprises a Management Team accountable to the Board of Governors (the Board itself comprises representatives of the therapy and fund-raising teams as well as senior professionals from health and educational fields), with Heads of Department based in London who represent the major operational areas of the charity: clinical services, training, research, national outreach and publicity. A team of seven Regional Heads, accountable to the Head of National Outreach, represent staff working at over 50 outreach locations nationwide.

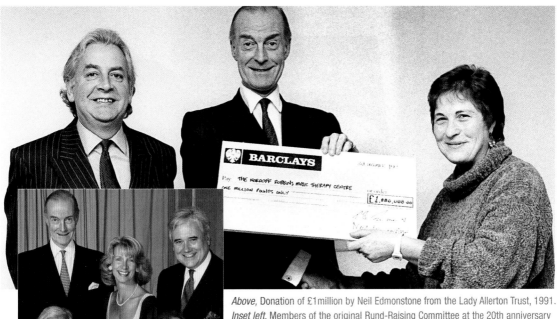

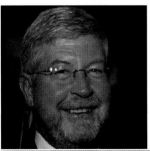

Above, Donation of £1million by Neil Edmonstone from the Lady Allerton Trust, 1991.
Inset left, Members of the original Rund-Raising Committee at the 20th anniversary
of the Silver Clef Lunch, 1995: clockwise from top left, Neil Edmonstone, Sam Alder,
Willie Robertson, Andrew Miller with Dee Dee Wilde.

Below, The Fund-Raising team, clockwise from top left, Audrey
Hoare, Director of Fund-Raising; Nicky Weller, Fund-Raising Manager;
Rachel Willmott and Gemma Fleet, Fund-Raising Assistants.

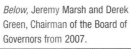

Left, Brian McLaughlin, Chairman
of the Fund-Raising Committee.

Below, Jeremy Marsh and Derek
Green, Chairman of the Board of
Governors from 2007.

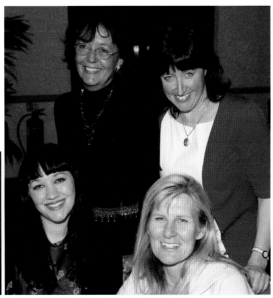

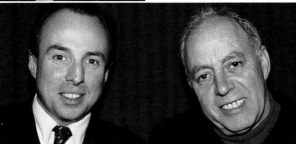

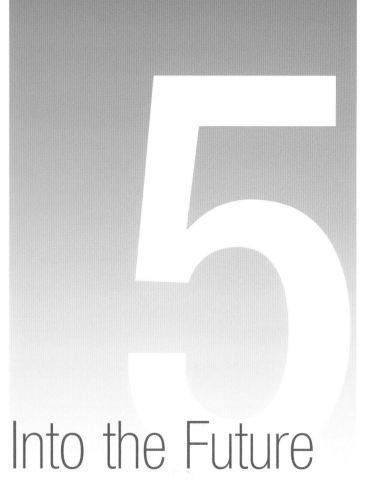

5

Into the Future

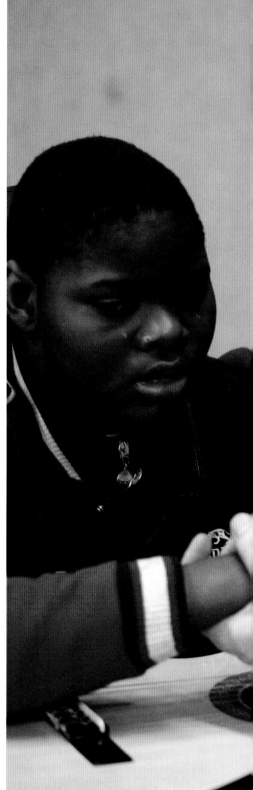

The focus in the early days of the Nordoff-Robbins charity was to establish a permanent clinic for the provision of music therapy and a secure foundation for the training of musicians to carry out the work. Once this had been achieved there was a natural desire to expand the provision of music therapy around the country; qualified therapists also began to take the work abroad.

In April 1995 the global composition of the Nordoff-Robbins community was celebrated by the First International Symposium of Nordoff-Robbins Music Therapists at the London Centre. This event honoured not only the international profile of Nordoff-Robbins practitioners, but also the progressive nature of the work in adapting itself to the needs of widely differing people and cultures. The success of the symposium was repeated in 2001 in New York and in 2006 in Germany.

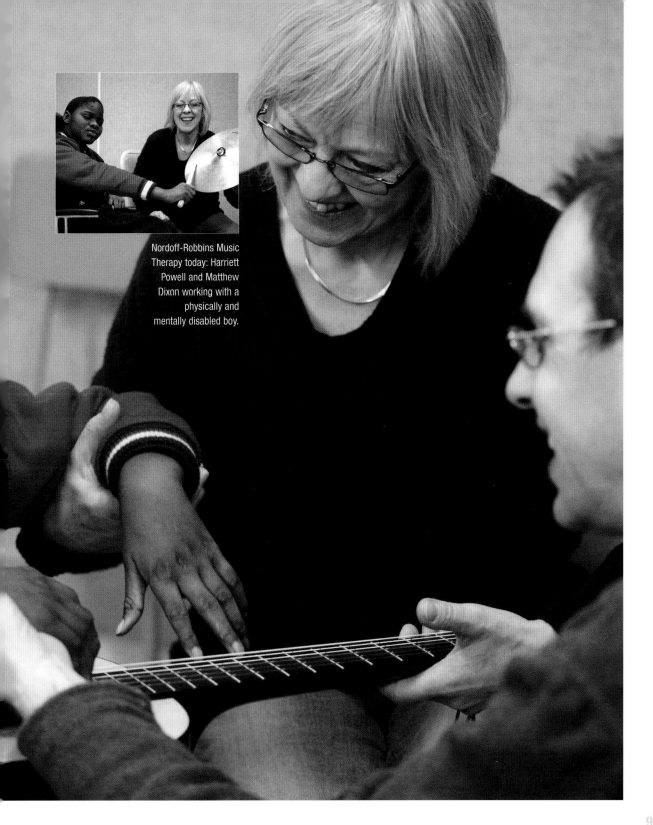

Nordoff-Robbins Music
Therapy today: Harriett
Powell and Matthew
Dixon working with a
physically and
mentally disabled boy.

This final chapter explores the spread of Nordoff-Robbins Music Therapy, the important role that London-trained therapists have played in this process, and the implications of these developments for the future of the charity.

Development of Nordoff-Robbins UK National Outreach

The funding of music therapists in venues around Britain is being developed comprehensively today in response to the dual need to serve a wider geographical area and to reach clients who, because of the nature of their disability or illness, cannot travel to the Centre easily. The benefits have been clear: as well as disseminating knowledge of the work, therapists can contribute more easily to multidisciplinary team-working in NHS services and schools, and have enhanced opportunities for clinical innovation.

From the earliest days at Goldie Leigh, Sybil Beresford-Peirse considered the secondment of therapists into schools an important adjunct to the work at a main Centre. This expanded in 1984 when Sybil agreed to support the department at Queen Mary's Hospital for Children in Surrey and, in 1989, the work of Colin Lee at London Lighthouse. However, it was under Pauline Etkin's leadership that outreach work blossomed. In 1994 Nicky O'Neill began an innovative secondment, one day a week, at Great Ormond Street Hospital, working with children with life-threatening illness in the Host Defence Directorate. This was followed by several projects set up to provide placement opportunities for the second-year students, coordinated by Rachel Verney.

Rachel Verney's appointment in 2002 as Outreach Coordinator (later Head of National Outreach) opened a new chapter in the development of Nordoff-Robbins-funded projects throughout the country, which in 2007 number over 50. Her long-term vision is to provide a network of regional Nordoff-Robbins Centres and projects throughout the country,

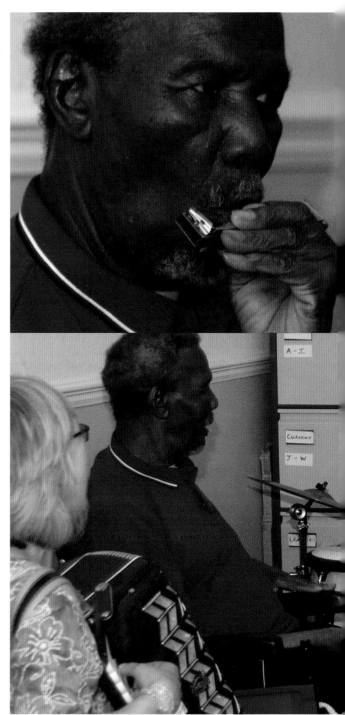

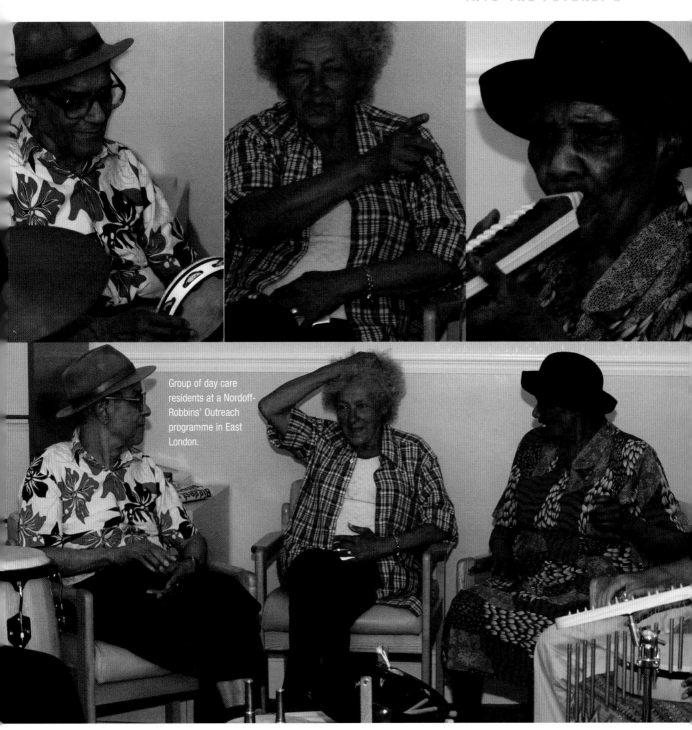

Group of day care residents at a Nordoff-Robbins' Outreach programme in East London.

the Centres being conceived as satellite centres that will facilitate the growth of music therapy in the local area. Three Centres have already been established: at Chetham's School of Music in Manchester, Mary Hare School for Deaf Children in Berkshire, and the BRIT School for Performing Arts and Technology in Croydon. The various smaller projects in host institutions comprise a mixture of fully funded and part-funded projects. In several instances a project has begun by being funded by Nordoff-Robbins, with internal support for the work gradually enabling funding to be taken over completely by the host institution.

The growth of the Nordoff-Robbins outreach programme has facilitated significant expansion of the variety of pathologies and conditions with which music therapists are working, as well as the settings in which they work. This has contributed to a broadening application of the core tenets of the Nordoff-Robbins approach. In particular the growth of Outreach is influenced by the community focus of Paul and Clive's early teamwork. Paul and Clive frequently saw children individually and in groups (often progressing from the former to the latter), along with larger-scale musical projects involving the whole school. These methods are closely related to the vision for Nordoff-Robbins that Rachel Verney sets out:

I would love to see a Nordoff-Robbins presence in as many institutions as possible. I would love to see it as little energy points, fermenting the life of music in and around the institution. Each unit will be like an *animateur*, both creating and serving the community that it is in.

Gary Ansdell used the term 'community music therapy' in his 2002 article 'Community Music Therapy and the Winds of Change' to describe this vision of music therapy. The essence of community music therapy is that it aims to work with people in *context*, acknowledging social and cultural factors of their health and illness, and reflecting the notion of music as a communal activity. Used in this way, music therapy has the power to *create* community, by bringing music to a group or institution.

Scotland

A Nordoff-Robbins presence in Scotland began to develop from the earliest days, when Julienne Cartwright moved to East Lothian in 1973 and pioneered the approach with adult clients. By 1983 she had been joined by five other Nordoff-Robbins-trained therapists: Elisabeth Blackwood, Mercédès

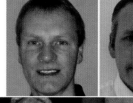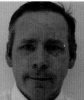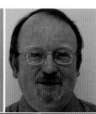

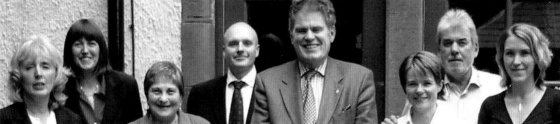

Board of Management, Scotland, *left to right*, James Robertson, MSc Programme Director, David Clement, Adminstrator and Company Secretary and Chris Achenbach Director of Services, 1998–2007. *Below*, left to right, Heather Gardner, Helen Patey, Pauline Etkin, Brian Fulton, John Ferguson-Smith (Chairman), Mary Brown, Co-Executive Director, Stuart Hornall and Janet Halton, Co-Executive Director.

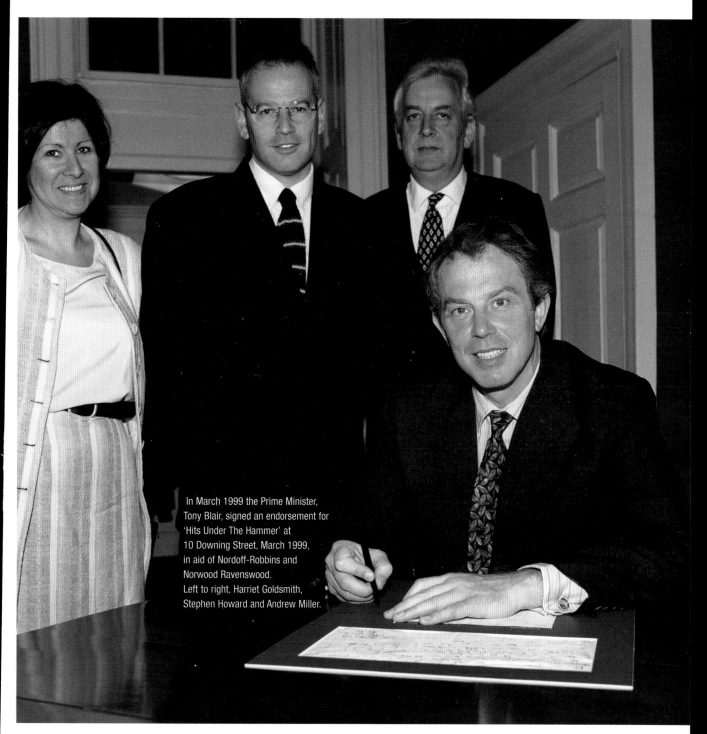

In March 1999 the Prime Minister,
Tony Blair, signed an endorsement for
'Hits Under The Hammer' at
10 Downing Street, March 1999,
in aid of Nordoff-Robbins and
Norwood Ravenswood.
Left to right, Harriet Goldsmith,
Stephen Howard and Andrew Miller.

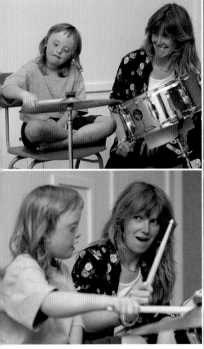

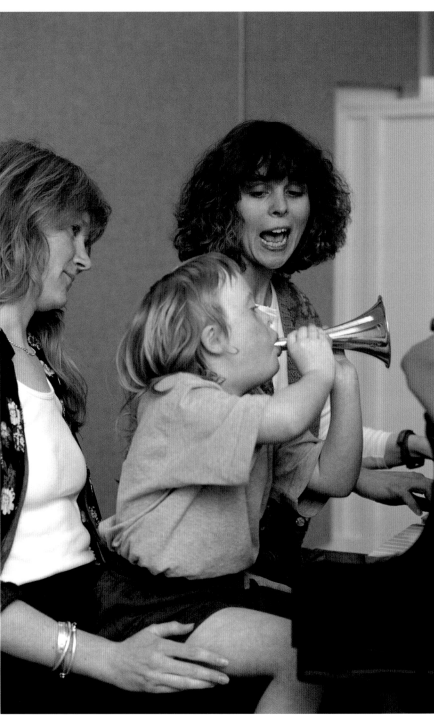

Jane Rous (top and middle left) and Lynda Byrt (main picture right) engage a young child with Down's Syndrome.

Pavlicevic (like Julienne, a South African national), Cressida Nash, April Parkins and James Robertson, who formed a close community of practitioners working with adults and children. With funding from several business charity events, including Sandy Irvine Robertson's Scottish Business Achievement Award luncheons, Nordoff-Robbins Scotland began to develop an independent identity. Public presentations were organised and a number of professionals in musical and health fields became interested in the work.

The need for research evidence was high on the agenda and the profile was raised, first in 1984, when Julienne Cartwright was awarded the Research Fellowship in Music Therapy at City University, London (a post established in 1981, supported by the Music Therapy Charity and Nordoff-Robbins Music Therapy), and then, in 1987, by Mercédès Pavlicevic's research grant from the Biomedical Committee of the Scottish Home and Health Department, which enabled her to undertake a PhD at Edinburgh University. Her successful completion of this in 1991 was a landmark achievement, being the first PhD awarded in the world to a Nordoff-Robbins-trained music therapist.

By this time the Nordoff-Robbins presence in Scotland had expanded still further with the arrival of Chris Achenbach, Felicity North, Caroline Boa, Steve Goodacre and Alyson Carter as Head and with the fund-raising support of Charles Barber, an Edinburgh-based management consultant. The Tartan Clef Awards were established as the charity's main annual event. Among the goals of the new charity was the establishment of a Nordoff-Robbins Unit in Scotland; this was realised in 1995, with the inauguration of a community-based service operating from an office at St Joseph's Hospital, Rosewell (just south of Edinburgh), where Nordoff-Robbins therapists had worked since Mercédès Pavlicevic first began in 1981. Without a training programme in operation there was no need for sizeable premises; instead, therapists went out from the Unit to undertake work in a variety of clinical settings. Work was also established further afield, in Glasgow and the surrounding area.

A Scottish training programme had been a dream of Alyson Carter's since she first arrived in Scotland in 1989. In 1997 detailed discussions were initiated with Neil Houston, a music lecturer at Moray House School of Education (then part of Heriot-Watt University), for the establishment of a Nordoff-Robbins training programme at the University. A syllabus based on the London training was approved in 2001 by the UK Council for Professions Supplementary to Medicine (forerunner of the Health Professions Council). The first Postgraduate Diploma Course in Music Therapy (Nordoff-Robbins) in Scotland began with five students in August 2002 at Moray House, which had merged with the University of Edinburgh's Department of Education in 1998 with James Robertson as Programme Coordinator, funded primarily by Nordoff-Robbins in London, with support from the Scottish charity and Moray House School of Education. In 2005 the programme converted to a two-year, full-time Master's degree (MSc) and moved to Queen Margaret University College in Edinburgh (becoming Queen Margaret University in 2007).

Today Nordoff-Robbins Music Therapy in Scotland employs 13 therapists and a full-time administrator. Chris Achenbach succeeded Alyson Carter as Head of Unit (Director of Services) in 1998 and the main office moved to Loanhead, Midlothian. In 2007 it moved a few miles to new premises in Lasswade. Today Chris continues to work for the charity but was succeeded in 2007 by two Co-Executive Directors, Mary Brown and Janet Halton. The charity has also been at the forefront of music therapy cross-fertilisation, employing music therapists from different UK training programmes. While retaining its status as an independent charity, with its own fund-raising committee under the chairmanship of Donald MacLeod, Nordoff-Robbins Music Therapy in Scotland is part-funded by the main UK Nordoff-Robbins charity, as is the training programme in Edinburgh.

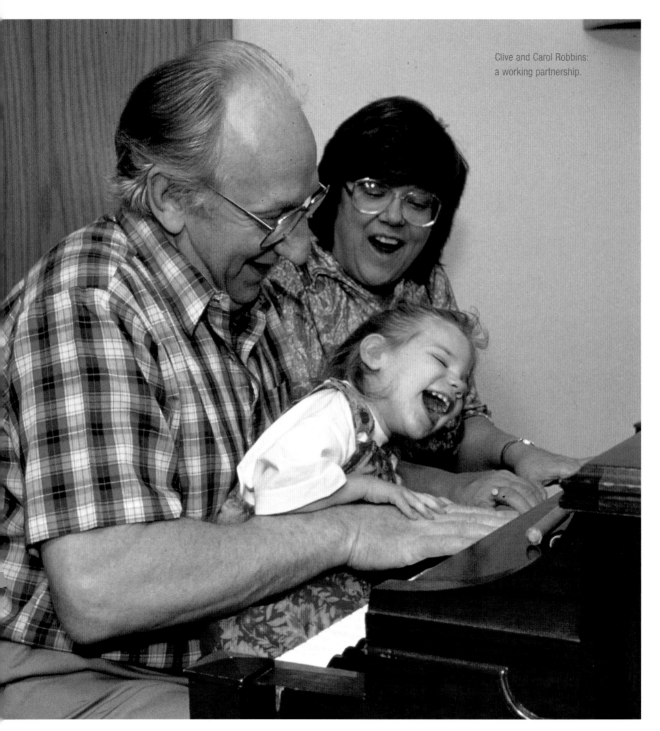

Clive and Carol Robbins:
a working partnership.

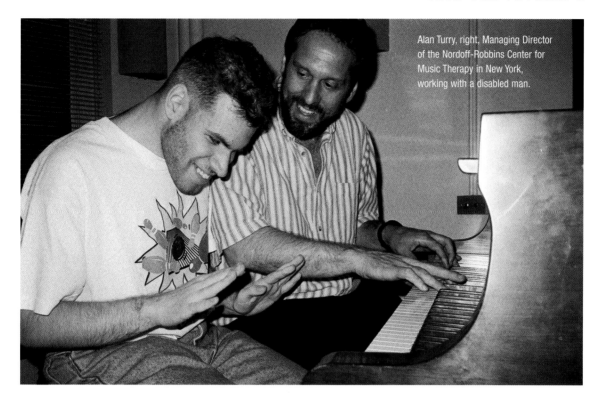

Alan Turry, right, Managing Director of the Nordoff-Robbins Center for Music Therapy in New York, working with a disabled man.

America

In 1961, after their pioneering experiments in England, Paul Nordoff and Clive Robbins settled in the USA for several years, establishing work initially in Pennsylvania. These years comprised a formative and highly fertile stage of their creative relationship and the consolidation of their working approach.

Clive returned to America in 1975 to marry his second wife, Carol, also a music therapist. A rewarding and productive partnership was formed, which saw them working first at the New York State School for the Deaf (1975–81), and then in Dallas, as Meadows Distinguished Visiting Professors of Music Therapy at Southern Methodist University (1981–82). They gave many lectures and summer courses and close contact was maintained in Europe with annual teaching engagements.

In 1990, after seven years living in Australia, Clive and Carol fulfilled a dream in their establishment of a Nordoff-Robbins Center for Music Therapy at New York University. From the academic side, this came about through the success of their summer courses at NYU and the enthusiasm of Professor Barbara Hesser, Director of NYU's Masters Music Therapy programme (Barbara herself had been trained by early students of Paul and Clive). The plan also had the strong support of Dean Jerrold Ross, Chairman of the Department of Music and Performing Arts Professions, and the President of the University, John Brademas. To finance the venture, the Nordoff-Robbins fund-raisers in London, Andrew Miller, Willie Robertson and Sam Alder, played a central role in founding the Nordoff-Robbins Music Therapy Foundation in America in September 1988. This organisation drew inspiration for its operational strategy directly from the London model and

Tom

Tom, a 79-year-old man, suffered from advanced Alzheimer's disease. His wife, herself becoming frail, had agreed reluctantly to his admission into a nursing home. In his youth Tom had drunk to excess and boxed; at first he had been in the army, but later in life had suffered many years of unemployment. Now, with increasing cognitive loss, he felt angry and desperate: like many of the residents in the nursing home, he did not understand why he was there, and he spent long periods at the front door, wrestling with the lock, inflamed by his loss of freedom. Not surprisingly, Tom was frequently quite violently abusive to staff and residents in the home.

A music therapist visited the home on a weekly basis and Tom was brought to see him. Their early sessions together were explosive, with Tom shouting and battering the percussion instruments as hard as he could, avoiding any contact and often storming out after five or ten minutes. The therapist continuously matched this huge energy with strong and forceful music at the piano. Over a period of months, Tom stayed longer in the room each week, and the music he made became gentler. He began to listen and respond to the therapist's music with answering phrases, and one week, when invited to sing a simple song about sharing, Tom joined in happily. Making music together enabled Tom and the therapist to connect with directness and implicit understanding; speech, which was increasingly difficult for Tom, was extraneous in this relationship.

The nursing staff at the home noticed that Tom's general level of desperation had begun to subside. He was less aggressive to others and easier to care for. Although he continued to be challenged by his condition, his behaviour indicated that he had begun to experience greater feelings of well-being and was more reconciled to his circumstances.

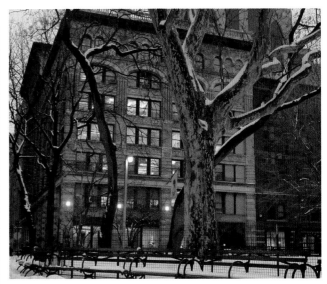

Steinhardt School of Culture, Education and Human Development, New York University, home of the Nordoff-Robbins Center for Music Therapy.

benefited from the support of many well-known musicians, as well as music business luminaries Ahmet Ertegün (1923–2006) who became Chairman and Ian Ralfini who became President with his wife Sunny as fund-raiser. The new Center served as both a clinical site and a training venue for music therapists in the Nordoff-Robbins approach, and in 1991 Kenneth Aigen's appointment as Director of Research at the Center facilitated the growth of a dynamic research profile (which was much needed).

Disaster struck in late 1995, when Carol was diagnosed with cancer of the gall bladder, and she died just over a year later in December 1996, at the age of 54. Shortly before her death, Carol was honoured, at a ceremony in New York, with a Silver Clef Award from the London charity, and a Foundation Award from the Nordoff-Robbins Foundation in America. A few days later she also received a Lifetime Achievement Award from the American Association for Music Therapy. The music therapy community worldwide united in testimony to the richness that she had brought to the profession. In 1997 Clive compiled an anthology of the worldwide messages of appreciation about Carol before and after her death, published under the title, *What a Wonderful Song Her Life Sang!* Many from England wrote of Carol's deep influence on their development during Clive and Carol's annual teaching visit to the London training programme.

Carol's death was a huge loss for Clive personally, but despite that he managed to continue his own commitment to the work. Today, in his 80th year, he is still writing, practising and teaching at the New York Center and internationally, particularly in the Far East, in partnership with his third wife, Kaoru Robbins. Day-to-day running of clinical services and the training programme was taken over in 1998 by Alan Turry and Ken Aigen on their appointment as Center Co-Directors, with Clive becoming Founding Director. The New York Center was to face further serious difficulties: the 9/11 terrorist attack on the World Trade Center had a paralyzing effect on fund-raising operations, while internal changes in the music industry resulted in serious setbacks in its support for the Foundation. At the time of writing the Foundation is regrouping after the death in 2006 of its Chairman, Ahmet Ertegün. The formation of a new board is underway with Clive as Chairman, and new fund-raising initiatives are being taken. The Center continues to operate as part of the Graduate Music Therapy programme at NYU, under the direction of Barbara Hesser, providing treatment for over 100 children, adolescents and adults weekly, and acting as a venue for training, research and learning. Following Ken Aigen's departure to direct the music therapy programme at Temple University, Alan Turry has become Managing Director of the Center, with Barbara Hesser as Director.

On the other side of the continent, 2006 saw the launch of Nordoff-Robbins Music Therapy West, with a publicity event in Los Angeles in March. An initial clinical project is up and running at the Music Therapy Wellness Clinic within California State University, Northridge.

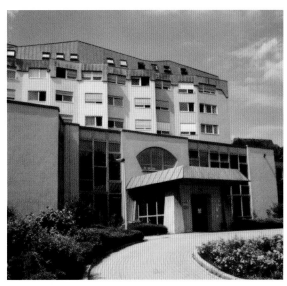

Herdecke Hospital, Cologne-Merheim, Köln, Germany.

Germany

It was in Germany that Paul Nordoff died in 1977, and the anthroposophical hospital where he chose to approach his final illness became the setting for a Nordoff-Robbins training programme the following year, 1978, which has continued to the present day. Established in 1969, the Gemeinnutziges-gemeinschafts Krankenhaus Herdecke in Germany's industrial Ruhr district was an innovative community hospital combining traditional and complementary medicine that aimed to foster physical, psychological and spiritual health. Nordoff greatly interested one of the hospital's founders, Dr Konrad Schily, in his work, and plans for a training programme were drawn up before Nordoff died.

The first programme in 1978 was ambitious in conception, aiming to inform students in both a psychoanalytic approach to music therapy and the Nordoff-Robbins approach, and also to qualify students to train others as music therapists. This two-year *mentoren* programme was led by Johannes Eschen,

President of the Deutsche Gesellschaft für Musiktherapie, who taught the psychoanalytic approach, and Merete Birkebæk and Rachel Verney, who had trained at Goldie Leigh and taught the Nordoff-Robbins approach. Clive and Carol Robbins were also involved as guest teachers. At the end of the course Johannes Eschen went on to Hamburg to establish psychoanalytic music therapy training there, while the Herdecke programme evolved into a Nordoff-Robbins training, initially with a one-year diploma programme under Merete Birkebæk's leadership.

In 1983 the Universität Witten-Herdecke opened as an adjunct to the hospital, and in 1985 an Institute for Music Therapy was established within the university. The training programme expanded into a two-year degree. Lutz Neugebauer, who trained with Sybil Beresford-Peirse (1981/82), succeeded Merete Birkebæk in 1988 as Co-Director of the Institute with Dagmar Gustorff, and became Director in 2002. Also in 1988 Professor David Aldridge was appointed Chair of Qualitative Research at the University, establishing a PhD programme, and has since made a major contribution to music therapy literature. At Witten-Herdecke research activity has flourished in many diverse areas of music therapy (including psychosomatic medicine, cancer treatment, dementia care, coma patients, psychiatry, pain management, HIV+ and AIDS): this reflects the hospital setting in which Nordoff-Robbins Music Therapy developed in Germany from the start, unlike England where the work developed for some years exclusively with children with disabilities.

The Institute for Music Therapy at Witten-Herdecke has grown to its present status through income generated by a fund-raising organisation, *Stiftung Nordoff-Robbins Musiktherapie*, which has paralleled the work of the Silver Clef committee in England, raising money through the rock music industry, with an annual fund-raising dinner since 1992 and other industry events.

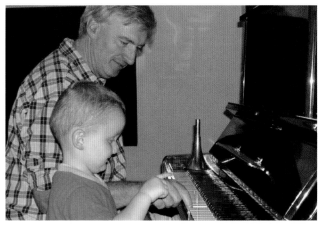

Robin Howat, Australia.

In 2005 Peter Hoffmann succeeded Lutz Neugebauer as Director of the Institute for Music Therapy and a new Nordoff-Robbins Therapy Clinical Centre was founded close to the University, co-directed by Lutz Neugebauer and David Aldridge and providing another venue for students' clinical training work.

Australia and New Zealand

In the summer of 1974, immediately after the completion of the first Goldie Leigh course, Paul and Clive undertook a successful lecture tour of Australia and New Zealand, at the invitation of Karl Kaltenbach, a pioneer of anthroposophical curative education in Australia. Enid Rowe heard them speak and, enthralled by their work, she subsequently went to London to undertake the Goldie Leigh training (1977/78). Returning to Sydney a year later, armed with her diploma, Enid was the first qualified Nordoff-Robbins therapist in Australia, and was to play a leading role in building up the Nordoff-Robbins establishment there.

Clive and Carol began to lecture in Australia from 1981 and made it their permanent home from 1984 to 1989, establishing a Nordoff-Robbins Music Therapy Centre at Warrah (where Karl and Hannelor Kaltenbach had founded their anthroposophical school) and a Nordoff-Robbins Association in Australia. After their return to the USA there was a strong desire to establish a Nordoff-Robbins training programme in Australia. Enid Rowe appealed to the international Nordoff-Robbins community for assistance and Robin Howat arrived in 1993, having been Head of Training in London for five years. The following year Enid and Robin began a one-year, full-time programme at Warrah, accredited by the Australian Music Therapy Association (AMTA), which ran successfully for three years. Sadly, lack of funds prevented the programme from continuing, although Robin and Enid maintained a modular course during the school holidays, as well as busy clinical practices.

Simultaneously, however, contact was established with the Golden Stave Foundation, an organisation that had been founded in 1978 by a group of music publishers in Sydney, who on hearing about the success of the Silver Clef Lunch in London wanted to do something similar, using the music industry as a vehicle for raising funds for charitable causes. At this time there were no Nordoff-

Golden Stave Music Therapy Centre, Sydney, Australia.

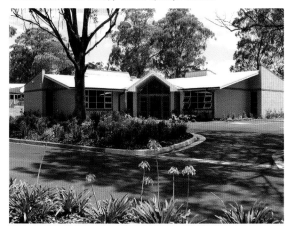

A Mother's Story

'Naomi was born with an extremely rare and degenerative syndrome. With her diagnosis came a long list of terrifying conditions that painted a very bleak picture, and seemed to deny the beauty of the adored baby in my arms. Most devastatingly, we were told that Naomi would not grow much bigger than a newborn baby, that she would be severely disabled physically and mentally, and would have a very short life.

Today Naomi is a beautiful seven-year-old, a tiny 14 pounds in weight, but with enormous spirit and personality. Although she is often ill, her spirit shines, and by a stroke of good luck we were introduced to Nordoff-Robbins three years ago. Naomi's music therapy sessions are a high point of her week and she has developed a trusting bond with her therapist. She loves to hear the greeting song that starts her session and her face is lit by a smile as she reaches out to touch the piano. She laughs as she tickles the skin of the drum, gently touches the chimes or purposefully lets a tambourine crash to the floor, waiting for a response.

I have had the privilege of sitting in these sessions, and have been amazed at the atmosphere and energy in the room. You might think that, for someone as small and frail as Naomi, a music therapist may simply soothe her with the most gentle of lullabies. But not so! With superb musical skill the therapist improvises gutsy, robust music that has Naomi laughing, clapping and stamping her feet. In music Naomi is well. Even on the darkest days, when Naomi is sick, her therapist will reach out to her and play music that hears her quietness, her stillness.

The benefits of music therapy spread like ripples in a pond. I leave the Nordoff-Robbins Centre in London each week with a brighter heart and a lighter step, and return to a happier home for our family. Whatever lies in store, in music therapy Naomi is celebrating her life with us all, and that is a rich and extraordinary experience.'

Robbins therapists in Australia, and the Golden Stave Foundation decided that it would raise money for ParaQuad, the Paraplegic and Quadraplegic Association, through various activities including an annual Golden Stave Lunch. In 1995 the Trustees began to work with Robin and Enid to establish a new Nordoff-Robbins Centre and institute a training course with proper academic credentials. A new charity, Nordoff-Robbins Music Therapy Australia Ltd (NRMTA), was incorporated in 1997, which became the Golden Stave Foundation's principal recipient. A close relationship was formed between the Trustees of the Golden Stave Foundation and the Directors of NRMTA, engineered particularly by Nick Hampton (and his wife Jean) who is a member of both Boards and who played a pivotal role throughout these developments.

The result of this generous backing was, first, the launch of a Graduate Diploma in Creative Music Therapy at the University of Western Sydney in March 2001, a two-year, part-time programme under the leadership of Robin Howat, accredited by AMTA. Second, the Golden Stave Music Therapy Centre, the first purpose-built music therapy centre in Australia, was built on the University campus and was formally opened on 1 November 2001 by Professor Marie Bashir, Governor of New South Wales, who later became the Centre's Official Patron. The Centre employs nine part-time therapists, who work in the Centre and in outreach programmes in children's hospital wards, special schools and aged care facilities. In 2004 a new Master's degree course was launched to replace the graduate diploma.

Clive Robbins, Pauline Etkin and Robin Howat have also been involved with a new venture in New Zealand: the opening in March 2004 of the Raukatauri Music Therapy Centre, the country's first ever music therapy centre (of which Robin Howat is a trustee). The Centre was the brainchild of New Zealander Hinewehi Mohi, a singer and songwriter, whose profoundly disabled daughter, Hineraukatauri, has

severe cerebral palsy and received music therapy at the Nordoff-Robbins Centre in London in 1999. From Hineraukatauri's lively response, Hinewehi and her husband George realised the need for a similar service back home, and together devoted themselves to the establishment of a centre, based on the principles of the Nordoff-Robbins approach, in Sandringham, Auckland. Establishing a charitable trust (the Raukatauri Music Therapy Trust) as a means of raising funds, with entertainment lawyer and artist manager Campbell Smith as Chair of the Trustees, they achieved success in attracting financial support from a number of organisations both within and outside the music industry. Some of New Zealand's best-known musicians, Bic and Boh Runga and Hayley Westenra, have acted as patrons. Yid-Ee Goh, who graduated from the London training in 2003, was employed at the Raukatauri Music Therapy Centre as its first therapist in 2004 and became Director in 2006.

South Africa

After completing her PhD at Edinburgh in 1991, Mercédès Pavlicevic returned to her native South Africa, where she spent the next three years developing a private practice in Johannesburg, with some funding support from the Nordoff-Robbins charity in London. Efforts were made to establish a fund-raising charity there, culminating in a large Silver Clef fund-raising ceremony in 1995, sponsored by EMI, which Pauline Etkin, Nancy Jarratt and Willie and Angi Robertson attended. A Silver Clef Award was presented at this event to a leading South African jazz musician, trumpeter Hugh Masekela. However, no permanent fund-raising organisation was established.

Mercédès was keen to start a training programme in music therapy, and with Kobie Temmingh, a colleague who had trained in the USA, she approached the music department of the University of Pretoria in 1997, with plans for a two-year

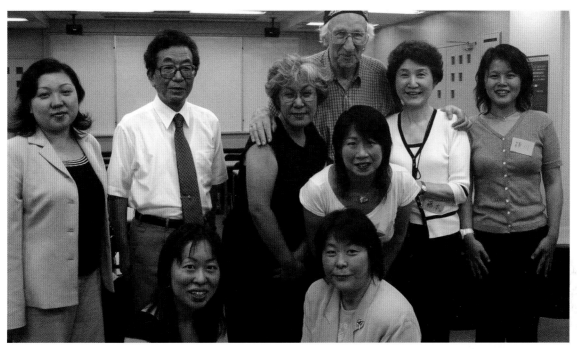

Clive with his wife Kaoru, centre, and members of the Organisation for the Study of Nordoff-Robbins Music Therapy (OSNRMT) in 2005, including graduates of Nordoff-Robbins training programmes in UK, US and Australia. Second left, Hiroko Fujimoto, co-founder of OSNRMT; second right, Professor Yohji Hayashi, translator of several Nordoff-Robbins texts.

Master's degree. The response was favourable and led to an initial intake of students in 1999, with the programme receiving formal validation by the Health Professions Council of South Africa in 2001. The Nordoff-Robbins curriculum document from London was used as a template, although the Pretoria training programme is not officially named Nordoff-Robbins because the University was unwilling to lay down such parameters. However, it closely parallels the London training in the organisation of modules, and Pauline Etkin and Gary Ansdell are its external examiners. Mercédès was offered a full-time position at the University in 2001 and was appointed to an Associate Professorship in 2002, a post she held until 2006 when she returned to London as Co-Head of Research. The Pretoria programme continues under the leadership of one of its graduates, Carol Lotter.

As elsewhere, the training programme is spawning the growth of music therapy in South Africa in a wide range of clinical areas. The work is developing its own national identity as it grows within the indigenous culture, drawing particularly on the time-honoured traditions of community music-making.

The Far East

Interest in music therapy grew in Japan from the 1950s and the country gained its first Nordoff-Robbins graduate in 1982 when Harumi Suzuki (née Koyama) completed the training programme in London. In 1984 Clive and Carol Robbins undertook a three-week lecture/workshop tour of several Japanese cities, at the invitation of the Anthroposophical Society in Japan, establishing permanent interest in the work.

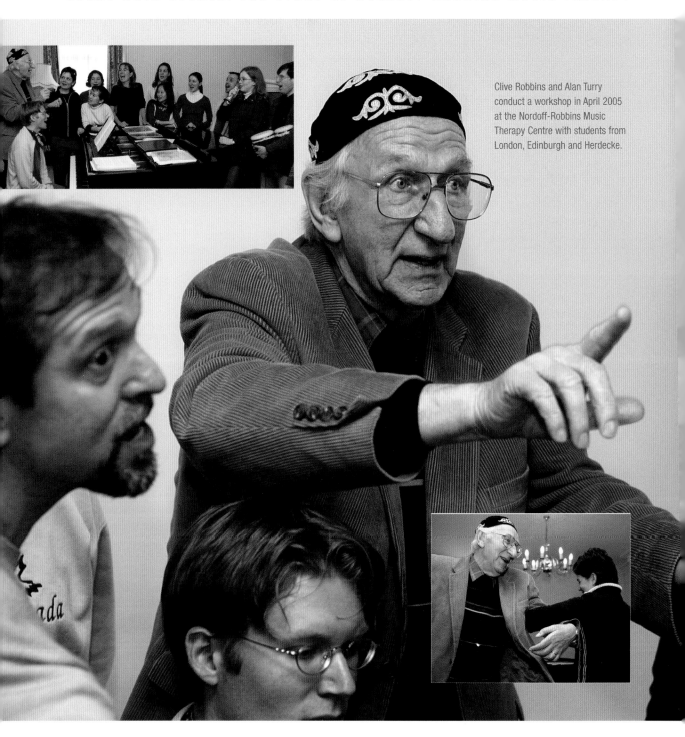

Clive Robbins and Alan Turry conduct a workshop in April 2005 at the Nordoff-Robbins Music Therapy Centre with students from London, Edinburgh and Herdecke.

In 1992 the Organisation for the Study of Nordoff-Robbins Music Therapy (OSNRMT) was founded in Tokyo by Hiroko and Atsushi Fujimoto, who had visited the Nordoff-Robbins Center for Music Therapy in New York. This organisation disseminates information about Nordoff-Robbins Music Therapy, through conferences, seminars, publications and translations of Nordoff-Robbins publications. A successful Clinical Supervision Program was instituted in 1999, in collaboration with the New York Center, coordinated by Kaoru Robbins (née Mochizuki) in New York, and administered in Japan by Harumi Suzuki and Noriko Hamatani, to fulfil some of the training and supervision needs of practitioners. Also involved with this venture, as a translator, was Kana Okazaki, who trained on the 1988/89 London programme, and later undertook doctoral studies at the New York Center.

From 1993 onwards Clive and Carol Robbins taught biannual summer courses in Japan. After Carol's death, Alan Turry and Ken Aigen joined Clive for these teaching excursions, which for several years became an annual event, attracting an average number of 400 participants. More recently, Clive was appointed Visiting Professor of Music Therapy from 2004-06 at the Senzoku Gakuen Music College, near Tokyo, and is the Honorary Director of the Music Therapy Institute at Senzuko. The work has spread widely in Japan, with graduates of four Nordoff-Robbins training programmes – England, the USA, Germany and Australia – and an OSNRMT membership of 235 at the time of writing.

Relations with the New York Center have also been established in Taiwan, Korea and China with invitations to lecture and teach. Clive is currently planning his fourth and fifth teaching visits to China, while several Koreans have graduated from the Nordoff-Robbins training programme in New York. Three Nordoff-Robbins graduates are teaching music therapy in Korean universities, while Ehwa Womans University in Korea has added a 'Nordoff-Robbins Component' to the University's music therapy training programme. There are active negotiations to implement Nordoff-Robbins training at Ewha and, in time, to establish a Nordoff-Robbins Centre.

Collaborative Partnerships

Today as Nordoff-Robbins UK faces the future, it does so with gratitude towards all that have made possible the outstanding work of the last 30 years. But the organisation also knows that it faces an uncertain future as there can be no complacent expectation that the £3 million raised each year from scratch will be sustained indefinitely. Though widely known, admired and supported, the charity cannot escape the fundamental fragility that underlies its existence. This is shared by Nordoff-Robbins establishments throughout the world and as a result the international Nordoff-Robbins community is striving towards greater unity and collaboration.

For example, the Scottish and English charities have become much more closely allied than they were initially, with members of the Scottish Board of Governors sitting on the English Board and vice versa. The same is true of the English and American charities, with some recent short-term financial support for the latter from London.

Within the English charity itself Pauline Etkin has, since becoming Managing Director, also fostered closer liaison between two sides of the charity – fund-raising and services – which were previously somewhat disconnected, surprising though this may seem. Envisioning the future of the charity involves a continual re-engagement between fund-raising and the three core elements of the charity's mandate – therapy, training and research – and a strategic plan that aims for collaborative effort both within and beyond the Nordoff-Robbins community.

The development of national outreach offers a potentially limitless expansion of service provision in partnership with institutions in education, health and social care, and in time

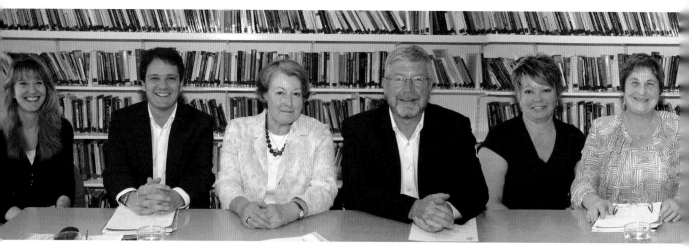

Board of Governors, 2006, comprised music therapy, fund-raising and senior allied health professional representatives.

Members present, left to right, Ruth Fluin-Hardy, Mike Miller, Nancy Jarratt, Brian McLaughlin, Prof. Jackie Campbell, Pauline Etkin,

the possibility of further training programmes with varying emphases; the research strategy also looks towards collaborative enquiry as a major strand of its rationale. The 30th year of the Nordoff-Robbins Charity's existence was one of the busiest and most successful. *A Year in the Life of Nordoff-Robbins* (see page 112) provides a brief insight into some of the important events in the charity's calendar, showing the range and scope of its various activities, as well as its growing international work.

The International Trust for Nordoff-Robbins Music Therapy

The International Trust for Nordoff-Robbins Music Therapy was formed in 1996, on the initiative of Pauline Etkin and Sam Alder, in order to preserve the name and reputation of Nordoff-Robbins and to hold the worldwide intellectual property assets of the work of Paul Nordoff and Clive Robbins. Six Trustees (later increased to eight) were appointed from

London and New York, representing the clinical and fund-raising aspects of the charities. A legal document was drawn up and signed by the Trustees which:

- preserves and protects archival material surviving from Nordoff and Robbins' original work;
- prevents misuse or unauthorised use of the name Nordoff-Robbins;
- preserves and protects the reputation of Nordoff-Robbins, ensuring that the high standard of care and treatment associated with the name are maintained;
- ensures that practitioners of Nordoff-Robbins Music Therapy receive adequate and proper training;
- ensures that the use of Nordoff-Robbins Music Therapy and associated training programmes throughout the world is governed and regulated;
- requires any individual or institution wishing to use the name of Nordoff-Robbins or the Silver Clef logo to seek permission to do so from the Trust.

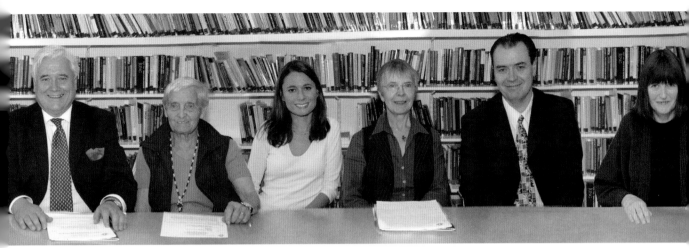

Sam Alder, Jean Eisler, Sophie Hampton (secretary), Sandra Brown, Dr Mark Morris and Helen Patey.

Members absent on this occasion, Hilary Came, Dr John Ferguson-Smith, Derek Green, Dr Clive Robbins and Willie Robertson.

The original Nordoff-Robbins archive material – recordings, notes and studies – as well as the right to approve use of the name Nordoff-Robbins have been assigned by Clive Robbins to the Trust. In addition, the Silver Clef logo, which is used extensively in fund-raising in the UK and the USA, is owned by the Trust.

The International Trust has generated criteria for the establishment of Nordoff-Robbins Centres, Units, Management Structures and training programmes, and provides permanent security that standards of practice associated with Nordoff-Robbins will be upheld rigorously.

From its humble origins at Sunfield, today Nordoff-Robbins Music Therapy is establishing itself as a fully national charity in the UK, while developments throughout the world promise significant expansion into the foreseeable future. In the words of Helen Patey, current President of the International Trust, 'We can be confident that wherever in the world the name of Nordoff-Robbins is used, the work will be of the highest quality, which is synonymous with the name.'

Many thousands of people have been drawn into the remarkable work of Nordoff-Robbins Music Therapy over the three decades of its existence. This book is a tribute to the countless children and adults who have changed their lives through music therapy, as well as parents and carers who have trusted and believed in the work; the founders of the approach, Paul Nordoff and Clive Robbins, for their pioneering zeal; the vision and determination of Sybil Beresford-Peirse, whose efforts resulted in the establishment of Nordoff-Robbins Music Therapy in London; the generations of music therapists, for their dedication to this noble work; the fund-raisers whose skill and commitment have financed the whole venture; and last but not least, the innumerable individuals who have been captivated by the possibilities of music therapy and given so generously – without them, quite simply, none of it would have happened.

2005/6 – A Year in the Life of Nordoff-Robbins

JUNE 05

The Silver Clef Lunch, sponsored by O₂, is the principal event in the fund-raising calendar with which the charity was launched in 1976. This month it celebrates its 30th anniversary with a ceremony attended by U2, The Who and others, raising a massive £700,000 for Nordoff-Robbins, around one quarter of the charity's annual income.

Sam Alder (Chair of the Board of Governors) is in Scotland for a meeting of the Scottish Charity Committee, while Pauline Etkin (Managing Director) meets with representatives of the BRIT School to discuss the building of a Nordoff-Robbins Unit on site.

Links with the wider music therapy profession continue to develop through the election of Helen Patey (Assistant Director) as Alternate Member of the Health Professions Council to represent Arts Therapists; Pauline Etkin as Education and Training Officer of the Association of Professional Music Therapists attends a meeting of Education Leads of the Allied Health Professions.

JULY

Nordoff-Robbins therapists speak regularly at national and international conferences about music therapy

Frances Murphy, Nordoff-Robbins Centre Receptionist since 1994.

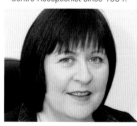

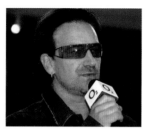

Bono at the 2005 Silver Clef Lunch where U2 received a Lifetime Achievement Award.

and related fields, and this month four members of the team fly to Australia to address the 11th World Congress of Music Therapy in Brisbane.

Marc Jaffrey, champion of the Music Manifesto initiative, visits the Nordoff-Robbins Centre. The Music Manifesto has been commissioned by the government to deliver improvements in the quality, depth and consistency of music education across the country and its aims, which include making every child's music matter and using the power of music to change lives, are strongly akin to those of music therapy. Discussions lead to Helen Patey signing the manifesto on behalf of the charity in June 2006.

AUGUST

At the Nordoff-Robbins Music Therapy Centre in London, a busy summer works programme is carried out to ensure that the fine buildings are kept in good repair. New facilities are provided for the growing collection of video and audio session recordings (all sessions are recorded and tapes must be stored confidentially).

Although sessions at the Centre take place only during school term-time, at National Outreach venues across

the country sessions continue through the summer, with hundreds of children and adults receiving music therapy each week. A current total of 33 music therapists are employed by the charity (part-time) working throughout the UK in seven geographical areas, each with its own regional Head. At this time Outreach projects number 42.

SEPTEMBER

Term begins for the new intake of students on the two Master's programmes in London and Edinburgh. The students in Edinburgh are the first group to undertake the new two-year MSc in Music Therapy at Queen Margaret University in Edinburgh which has grown out of the diploma programme established in 2002.

In London other educational opportunities run alongside the main training programme, including a ten-week improvisation course which also begins at the start of the academic term. Meanwhile staff preview a new promotional DVD commissioned by the Charity.

As National Outreach venues continue to increase and develop, Pauline Etkin this month visits new Nordoff-Robbins units at Chetham's School of Music in Manchester and Mary Hare School for Deaf Children in Berkshire, as well as a new project in Belfast. Rachel Verney (Head of National Outreach) appoints music therapist Harriet Crawford as her deputy.

OCTOBER

The biennial charity Strategy Meeting takes place at Highgate Golf Club, attended by representatives of the Board of Governors and the Fund-Raising Committee, Heads of Department and representatives of

the Scottish Charity including the Fund-Raising Chairman. This provides an opportunity to plan the future of the charity and review the strategic plan for Nordoff-Robbins service provision and fund-raising to grow by 10% per annum over the current five year period.

Pauline Etkin and Sam Alder visit the New York Center to review the partnership between the Nordoff-Robbins Music Therapy Foundation, Inc. and New York University.

Elsewhere in the UK a celebration marks the official launch of fund-raising in Manchester, while Nordoff-Robbins presents a one-day conference jointly with Mary Hare School and The Ear Foundation in Nottingham.

NOVEMBER

A busy month for fund-raising sees the Music Industry Trusts' Dinner, attended by Peter Gabriel, raise £179,000, the Woman of the Year Awards raise £22,000, the Proper Music Pop Quiz raise £17,000 and the Wimbledon Tennis Tournament raise £33,000, all for Nordoff-Robbins.

International links are also dynamic: Nordoff-Robbins Scotland celebrates its tenth birthday with a large cele-bration (the night before the annual Tartan Clef Awards); Pauline Etkin is in South Africa as external examiner for the Pretoria training programme (a role shared with Gary Ansdell); Gary Ansdell and Mercédès Pavlicevic host an International Research Symposium in collaboration with universities in Norway and South Africa; Sam Alder and Willie Robertson fly to Los Angeles to plan for the establishment of Nordoff-Robbins there.

Following successful viva examinations in October, graduating students from the training programme in London receive their Master's degrees at the Graduation Ceremony at the Nordoff-Robbins Centre.

DECEMBER

The third in a series of Continuing Education events organized by Donald Wetherick is held at the Centre, aimed at qualified members of the music therapy profession (the Health Professions Council requires every music therapist to complete mandatory Continuing Professional Development hours each year).

Helen Patey visits Bristol as external examiner for the music therapy training course at the University of Bristol. She is one of several Nordoff-Robbins therapists who take on this role for other therapy trainings (music and other arts), including Pauline Etkin, Gary Ansdell and Judith Nockolds.

The Nordoff-Robbins Carol Service is held at St Luke's Church, Chelsea with celebrity performers Joss Stone, The Choirboys, G4, Natasha Kaplinsky and others, raising £64,000 for the charity.

JANUARY 06

The new MPhil/PhD programme offered by the Nordoff-Robbins Charity, in partnership with City University, is launched. This has been a key target of the Research Department since its foundation in 2002, and ensures that the Centre's position as an international centre of excellence in music therapy training and research is maintained.

A group of visitors are welcomed at the Centre from Norway, led by Tom Naess who trained at Goldie Leigh in 1974. They are among many people interested or involved in music therapy who come to see the work of the Centre first hand.

Demand for more public knowledge about music therapy continues to be

met at the Centre, through a repetition of the ten-week improvisation course, as well as a ten-week 'Introduction to Music Therapy' course, both of which begin this month.

FEBRUARY

The annual BRIT Awards are held at Earl's Court, one of the major events in Britain's rock music calendar. Hosted by Chris Evans, there are prizes for Coldplay, Kaiser Chiefs, Paul Weller and others. Nordoff-Robbins receives £250,000 from the evening.

The British Society for Music Therapy holds one of it regular one-day conferences at the Centre, this one entitled 'Music Therapy and Families'.

MARCH

Preparations for selecting the next group of students to begin the two-year training programme are underway in London. Judith Nockolds (Year Two Co-ordinator of the training programme and Chair of the Association of Professional Music Therapists) leads an Open Evening for musicians interested in undertaking the programme, while auditions coordinated by Sandra Brown take place for the six available places. The British Society for Music Therapy also holds an Introductory Day at the Centre for people interested in music therapy.

Rachel Verney coordinates an Outreach Day at the Centre for therapists working in outreach projects across the UK. Many work in relative professional isolation and opportunities to meet together are rare.

Three events on different days maintain the Continuing Education series for music therapists on varied topics: music in physiotherapy, music in speech and language therapy and music therapy with people with multiple sensory impairments.

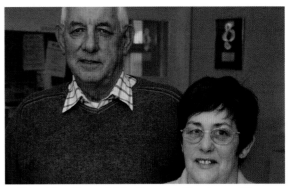

Mick and Rose Conway, Building Manager and Housekeeper of the Nordoff-Robbins Centre since 1995.

APRIL

Alan Turry, Director of the Nordoff-Robbins Center for Music Therapy in New York, makes his annual visit to London to spend a week with students on the training programme. This coincides with the annual meeting of the International Trust for Nordoff-Robbins Music Therapy (established 1996). On the agenda are: (1) criteria for the establishment of Nordoff-Robbins programmes worldwide; (2) copyright of intellectual property of Nordoff-Robbins; (3) funding of international Nordoff-Robbins centres in the UK, USA, Germany and Australia.

Fund-raising events continue with the HMV Football Extravaganza, an annual dinner for over 1000 people honouring football and footballers at the Grosvenor House Hotel. Hosted by Richard Keys, this year's dinner pays tribute to Alan Shearer and raises £608,000 for Nordoff-Robbins. Later in the month another long-established event, the Sandown Park Race Day in aid of Nordoff-Robbins raises a further £64,000.

MAY

Rachel Verney hosts an Outreach Celebration Day at the Centre to honour five years of Nordoff-Robbins outreach. The event is attended by over 100 representatives of Nordoff-Robbins partner organizations in

Health, Social Care and Education, providing an opportunity for them to learn about the Nordoff-Robbins outreach network and the contribution of music therapy to their organisations.

Visitors to the Centre this month include 30 music therapy students from Anglia Ruskin University, and representatives of local schools sending pupils for music therapy, who come to attend the biennial Headteachers' Meeting.

Year Two students make the Final Clinical Presentations of their training programme, an event followed by a meeting of the City University Board of Studies.

Final preparations are underway for the Third Nordoff-Robbins International Symposium held in Germany the following month (an event occuring every five years).

Arnold Johnson, Nordoff-Robbins Centre Technician since 1989.

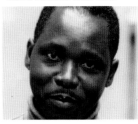

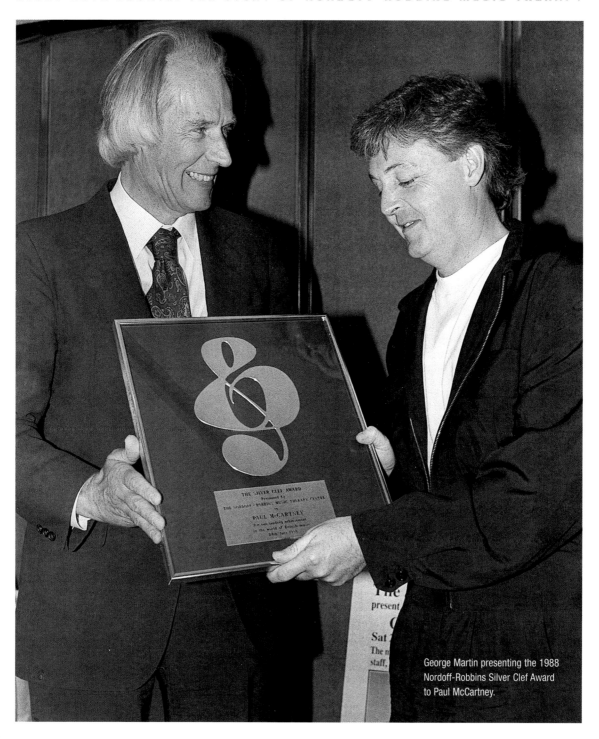

George Martin presenting the 1988 Nordoff-Robbins Silver Clef Award to Paul McCartney.

HONOURS*LIST*
SILVER CLEF AWARD WINNERS
1976-2006

These major artists have something important besides music. They are all winners of awards given by Nordoff-Robbins for outstanding services to the British music industry. All of these artists, who have learned the value of music therapy at first hand, join together in requesting your support for such a worthy cause which is entirely dependant on voluntary contributions.

SILVER CLEF LIFETIME ACHIEVEMENT AWARD
2006 The Eagles
2005 U2

SILVER CLEF AWARD
2006 Sharon & Ozzy Osbourne
2004 Morrissey
2003 Coldplay
2002 Dido
2001 Tom Jones
2000 Eurythmics
1999 M People
1998 Jamiroquai
1997 Elvis Costello
1996 Wet Wet Wet
1995 Take That
1994 Sting
1993 Eric Clapton
1992 Def Leppard
1991 Rod Stewart
1990 Robert Plant
1989 George Michael
1988 Paul McCartney
1987 David Bowie
1986 Phil Collins
1985 Dire Straits
1984 Queen
1983 Eric Clapton
1982 The Rolling Stones
1981 Status Quo
1980 Pink Floyd
1979 Elton John
1978 Genesis
1977 Cliff Richard & The Shadows
1976 The Who

NEW MUSIC AWARD
2006 Editors
2005 McFly (pop)
2005 Razorlight (rock)
2004 Jamie Cullum
2003 Ms Dynamite
2002 Blue
2001 Craig David
2000 Five
1999 Another Level
1998 Robbie Williams
1997 Kula Shaker
1996 Supergrass
1995 Eternal
1994 Dina Carroll
1993 Take That
1992 Right Said Fred
1991 James
1990 Lisa Stansfield
1989 Fairground Attraction
1988 Wet Wet Wet
1987 Pet Shop Boys
1986 Curiosity Killed The Cat

SPECIAL ACHIEVEMENT
2004 Iron Maiden
2003 Ray Davies
2002 Lulu
2001 Leiber & Stoller
2000 Bacharach & David
1999 Pete King
1998 Deep Purple
1997 Chris Barber
1995 George Martin
1993 The Bee Gees
1992 Alan Freeman

INTERNATIONAL AWARD
2006 Foo Fighters
2005 Sir Bob Geldof
2004 George Benson
2003 Bon Jovi
2002 Natalie Imbruglia
2001 Kylie Minogue
2000 Ronan Keating
1999 The Corrs
1998 Chris de Burgh
1997 Vanessa Mae
1996 AC DC
1995 Bryan Adams
1994 Jimmy Page & Robert Plant
1993 U2
1992 INXS

HEART 106.2 AWARD
2006 Girls Aloud
2005 Natasha Bedingfield
2005 Lemar
2004 Will Young
2003 Atomic Kitten
Additional Awards
30th Anniversary Award
2005 The Who

CLASSICAL AWARD
2006 Bryn Terfel
2005 Katherine Jenkins

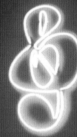

NORDOFF-ROBBINS
MUSIC THERAPY

ADDITIONAL AWARDS

30TH ANNIVERSARY AWARD
2005 The Who

BEST BRITISH GROUP AWARD
2006 Kaiser Chiefs

SILVER ACCOLADE AWARD
1999 Madness
1998 Sir Cliff Richard

WORLD PEACE AWARD
1997 John Lennon

2007 AWARDS

SILVER CLEF	Paul Weller
NEW MUSIC	Paulo Nutini
INTERNATIONAL	John Legend
HEART 106.2	The Feeling
CLASSICAL	Andrea Bocelli
BEST BRITISH GROUP	Snow Patrol
ICON	Rod Stewart
AMBASSADORS OF ROCK	Bryan Ferry

Select Bibliography

For an exhaustive list of books and articles published by researchers and practitioners of Nordoff-Robbins Music Therapy, the reader is recommended to visit the website of the New York Center for Nordoff-Robbins Music Therapy:

www.nyu.edu/education/music/nrobbins

and follow the links for publications

Aigen, K. (1996) *Being in Music: Foundations of Nordoff-Robbins Music Therapy,* Nordoff-Robbins Music Therapy Monograph Series, Volume 1. St Louis, MO: MMB Music, Inc.

Aigen, K. (1998) *Paths of Development in Nordoff-Robbins Music Therapy.* Gilsum, NH: Barcelona Publishers.

Aigen, K. (2005) *Music-centered Music Therapy.* Gilsum, NH: Barcelona Publishers.

Ansdell, G. (1995) *Music for Life. Aspects of Creative Music Therapy with Adult Clients.* London: Jessica Kingsley Publishers.

Lee, C. (2003) *The Architecture of Aesthetic Music Therapy.* Gilsum, NH: Barcelona Publishers.

Nordoff, P. and Robbins, C. (1971) *Therapy in Music for Handicapped Children.* London: Gollancz. Republished (2004) Gilsum, NH: Barcelona Publishers.

Nordoff, P. and Robbins, C. (1971, 1983). *Music Therapy in Special Education.* St Louis, MO: MMB Music, Inc.

Nordoff, P. and Robbins, C. (1977) *Creative Music Therapy.* New York: John Day Company. 2nd ed. (2007) Gilsum, NH: Barcelona Publishers.

Patey, H. and Darnley-Smith, R. (2003) *Music Therapy.* London: Sage Publications Ltd.

Pavlicevic, M. (1997) *Music Therapy in Context: Music, Meaning and Relationship.* London: Jessica Kingsley Publishers.

Pavlicevic, M. and Ansdell, G. (eds) (2004) *Community Music Therapy.* London: Jessica Kingsley Publishers.

Robbins, C. and Robbins, C. (1980) *Music Therapy for the Hearing-impaired and Other Special Groups.* St Louis, MO: MMB Music, Inc.

Robbins, C. and Robbins, C. (eds) (1998) *Healing Heritage: Paul Nordoff Exploring the Tonal Language of Music.* Gilsum, NH: Barcelona Publishers.

Robbins, C. (2005) *A Journey into Creative Music Therapy.* Nordoff-Robbins Music Therapy Monograph Series, Volume 3. St Louis, MO: MMB Music, Inc.. Gilsum, NH: Barcelona Publishers.

Contacts

England

SERVICES

Nordoff-Robbins Music Therapy Centre
2 Lissenden Gardens
London NW5 1PQ
Tel: +44 (0)20 7267 4496
Fax: +44 (0)20 7267 4369
Email: admin@nordoff-robbins.org.uk
Web: www.nordoff-robbins.org.uk

FUND-RAISING

Fund-Raising Office
Nordoff-Robbins Music Therapy
Studio A2
1927 Building
2 Michael Road
London SW6 2AD
Tel: +44 (0)20 7371 8404
Fax: +44 (0)20 7371 8206
Email: admin@nrfr.co.uk

Scotland

SERVICES

Nordoff-Robbins Music Therapy in Scotland
Unit 2, Poltonhall Industrial Estate
Lasswade, Midlothian EH18 1BW
Tel: +44 (0) 13 1663 0033
Fax: +44 (0) 13 1663 0222
Email: davidclement@nrscot.org.uk
Web: www.nordoff-
robbins.org.uk/html/NR_Scotland.html

FUND-RAISING

Fund-Raising Coordinator
21 Sandyford Place
Glasgow G3 7NG
Tel: +44 (0)141 248 7548
Fax: +44 (0)141 248 7648
Email: nordoff-
robbins@scottishfundraising.fsnet.co.uk

USA

SERVICES/FUND-RAISING

Nordoff-Robbins Center for Music Therapy
New York University
82 Washington Square East, 4th Floor
New York
NY 10003
Tel: +1 (212) 998 5151
Fax: +1 (212) 995 4045
Email: nordoff.robbins@nyu.edu
Web: www.nyu.edu/education/music/nrobbins
Web: www.nordoffrobbins.org

Australia

SERVICES

Golden Stave Music Therapy Centre
University of Western Sydney
Building E, Second Ave
Kingswood
NSW 1797
Tel: +61 (0) 2 47 360 240
Fax: +61 (0) 47 360 211
Email: musictherapy@uws.edu.au
Web: www.nordoff-robbins.com.au

FUND-RAISING

Nordoff-Robbins Music Therapy Australia Ltd
Locked Bag 1797
Penrith South DC
NSW 1797
Tel: +61 (0) 2 9686 1277
Fax: +61 (0) 2 9686 1477
Email: nicci.nordoff-robbins@tpg.com.au

Germany

SERVICES/FUND-RAISING

Nordoff Robbins Zentrum Witten
Fördergesellschaft für Musiktherapie in Witten
und Umgebung e.V.
Ruhrstrasse 70
58452 Witten
Deutschland
Tel: +49 (0) 2302 282470
Email: info@nordoff-robbins.org
Web: nordoff-robbins.org

Index